AMA
GUIDELINES
FOR
ADOLESCENT
PREVENTIVE
SERVICES
(GAPS)

RECOMMENDATIONS
AND
RATIONALE

AMA
GUIDELINES
FOR
ADOLESCENT
PREVENTIVE
SERVICES
(GAPS)

RECOMMENDATIONS

AND

RATIONALE

•

ARTHUR B. ELSTER, M.D.
NAOMI J. KUZNETS, PH.D.

American Medical Association
Department of Adolescent Health
Chicago, Illinois

SANS TACHE

Williams & Wilkins

BALTIMORE • PHILADELPHIA • HONG KONG
LONDON • MUNICH • SYDNEY • TOKYO

A WAVERLY COMPANY

Editor: David C. Retford
Managing Editor: Molly L. Mullen
Copy Editor: Robert S. Winkler
Designer: Norman W. Och
Illustration Planner: Ray Lowman
Production Coordinator: Barbara J. Felton

Williams & Wilkins

BALTIMORE • PHILADELPHIA • HONG KONG
LONDON • MUNICH • SYDNEY • TOKYO

A WAVERLY COMPANY

Copyright © 1994
American Medical Association
515 North State Street
Chicago, Illinois 60610

Printed in the United States of America

Library of Congress Cataloging-in-Publication Data

American Medical Association.
 AMA Guidelines for adolescent preventive services (GAPS) recommendations and rationale / [edited by] Arthur Elster.
  p. cm.
 Includes bibliographical references and index.
 ISBN 0-683-02798-0
  1. Preventive health services for teenagers—United States—Standards. I. Elster, Arthur B. II. Title.
[DNLM: 1. Preventive Health Services—standards. 2. Adolescent Medicine—standards. 3. Delivery of Health Care—Standards. WS 460 A512a 1994]
RJ102.A42 1994
362.1'0835—dc20
DNLM/DLC
for Library of Congress
                                              93-4701
                                             CIP

                                95 96 97
                  3 4 5 6 7 8 9 10

For over 25 years, a special group of physicians, psychologists, nurses, nutritionists, health educators, and social and behavioral science researchers has worked to improve the health and well-being of adolescents. The efforts and achievements of these people provided the scientific and experiential beacon that culminated in the development of GAPS. We wish to dedicate this book to these professionals, both past and present, and to the adolescents for "whom the bells toll."

Table of Contents

Foreword

The publication of the American Medical Association's *Guidelines for Adolescent Preventive Services: Recommendations and Rationale* represents a landmark in adolescent health care. Developed by the American Medical Association with the assistance of a national scientific advisory board, Guidelines for Adolescent Preventive Services (GAPS) provides, for the first time, national systematically developed recommendations for delivering comprehensive adolescent clinical preventive services.

The continued decline in the health status of our adolescents requires that we undertake a fundamental restructuring of our approach to adolescent health care. Adolescent health research tells us that the greatest health threats for adolescents today are behavioral rather than biomedical, that adolescents engage in health behaviors at increasingly earlier ages, and that most youth engage in some type of personal behavior that threatens their health and well-being. Accordingly, GAPS recommends that, in addition to treating physical disease and the medical consequences of adolescent health risk behaviors, primary care providers should work to prevent or modify these behaviors.

GAPS provides a framework for the organization and content of routine health care for adolescents. Its recommendations address the system of health care delivery, the use of health guidance, the value of screening, and the need for immunizations. While preventive service schedules have been in place quite some time for infants and toddlers, we have had a void of guidance for adolescent preventive health care. GAPS recommends annual preventive service visits for adolescents which focus on health guidance, immunizations, and screening for physical, emotional, and behavioral conditions.

GAPS also stresses that adolescent health care delivery depends on a partnership in health promotion and disease prevention among parents, adolescents, and primary care providers. It includes recommendations for health guidance for families of adolescents, recognizing that parents need guidance in meeting the unique physical and emotional needs of their adolescents.

Special appreciation goes to Janet E. Gans, Ph.D., and Patricia B. Levenberg, Ph.D., who helped write and edit various sections of the book; to Beth Alexander, M.D., who helped write a section on reimbursement; to Kelly Towey for her overall technical assistance; to Robert C. Rinaldi, Ph.D., Director of the AMA's Division of Health Science, for his continued support of the GAPS project; to Lloyd Kolbe, Ph.D., and Mary Vernon, M.D., of the CDC for their vision and advice throughout the development of GAPS; and to many other AMA staff members who helped make this book possible.

Graphics Design (Chicago): Gregory Chambers

The authors wish to express their appreciation to the following people who reviewed chapters for this book:

Vincent A. Fulginiti, M.D.

Thomas Houston, M.D.

Marc S. Jacobson, M.D.

Michael D. Klitzner, Ph.D.

Barbara Long, M.D.

Donald P. Orr, M.D.

Anne C. Petersen, Ph.D.

John Santelli, M.D., M.P.H.

John Schowalter, M.D.

Mary Story, Ph.D.

Katherine Voegtle, Ph.D.

Esther Wender, M.D.

A list of additional people who reviewed material and helped formulate the GAPS recommendations can be found in *Guidelines for Adolescent Preventive Services,* a monograph published by the AMA, Department of Adolescent Health.

Financial support for GAPS was provided through Grant U63-CCU503075-01 from the Division of Adolescent and School Health, National Center for Chronic Disease Prevention and Health Promotion, Centers for Disease Control and Prevention.

Foreword

The publication of the American Medical Association's *Guidelines for Adolescent Preventive Services: Recommendations and Rationale* represents a landmark in adolescent health care. Developed by the American Medical Association with the assistance of a national scientific advisory board, Guidelines for Adolescent Preventive Services (GAPS) provides, for the first time, national systematically developed recommendations for delivering comprehensive adolescent clinical preventive services.

The continued decline in the health status of our adolescents requires that we undertake a fundamental restructuring of our approach to adolescent health care. Adolescent health research tells us that the greatest health threats for adolescents today are behavioral rather than biomedical, that adolescents engage in health behaviors at increasingly earlier ages, and that most youth engage in some type of personal behavior that threatens their health and well-being. Accordingly, GAPS recommends that, in addition to treating physical disease and the medical consequences of adolescent health risk behaviors, primary care providers should work to prevent or modify these behaviors.

GAPS provides a framework for the organization and content of routine health care for adolescents. Its recommendations address the system of health care delivery, the use of health guidance, the value of screening, and the need for immunizations. While preventive service schedules have been in place quite some time for infants and toddlers, we have had a void of guidance for adolescent preventive health care. GAPS recommends annual preventive service visits for adolescents which focus on health guidance, immunizations, and screening for physical, emotional, and behavioral conditions.

GAPS also stresses that adolescent health care delivery depends on a partnership in health promotion and disease prevention among parents, adolescents, and primary care providers. It includes recommendations for health guidance for families of adolescents, recognizing that parents need guidance in meeting the unique physical and emotional needs of their adolescents.

The new territory forged by these guidelines must be followed by the broad-based professional partnerships required for successful implementation. We must get beyond the traditional and categorical ways of designing and delivering health, education, and social services and bring together our expertise and resources to focus on the issues and problems facing adolescents. If we are to become genuinely responsive to the health and developmental needs of our adolescents, we must be driven by the adolescent as a whole and find new and better ways to link our disciplines, funding streams, and institutions. Adolescents need to receive coordinated health care and hear consistent health messages.

GAPS provides us a focal point for adolescent preventive health care through its recommendations which are based on a rigorous review of the evidence. I commend the Centers for Disease Control and Prevention and the American Medical Association for their leadership in the development of these guidelines.

We have no leadership without vision. With vision, we can build bridges from the present to the future. GAPS offers a clear vision of what adolescent health promotion and disease prevention should be. We now must build the bridges.

M. Joycelyn Elders, M.D.
U.S. Surgeon General

Acknowledgments

Members of the GAPS National Scientific Advisory Board:

Susan G. Millstein, Ph.D.
(Co-chair)
University of California, San Francisco

Jonathan D. Klein, M.D., M.P.H.
(Secretary)
University of Rochester

Alfred O. Berg, M.D.
American Academy of Family Physicians

Robert W. Blum, M.D., Ph.D.
University of Minnesota

Lawrence D'Angelo, M.D.
American College of Physicians

A. Robert Davies, M.S.
Nationwide Insurance

E. Harvey Estes, Jr., M.D.
AMA Council on Scientific Affairs

Brian R. Flay, D. Phil.
University of Illinois, Chicago

Phillip J. Goldstein, M.D.
American College of Obstetricians and Gynecologists

Michael D. Klitzner, Ph.D.
Pacific Institute

James F. Leckman, M.D.
American Psychiatric Association

Andrea Marks, M.D.
Society for Adolescent Medicine

Dan R. Offord, M.D.
Chedoke-McMaster Hospital

Guy S. Parcel, Ph.D.
University of Texas, Houston

Anne C. Petersen, Ph.D.
University of Minnesota

Joe M. Sanders, Jr., M.D.
American Academy of Pediatrics

John E. Schowalter, M.D.
American Academy of Child and Adolescent Psychiatry

Howard Schubiner, M.D.
Wayne State University

Richard M. Steinhilber, M.D.
AMA Council on Scientific Affairs

AMA Staff:
Arthur B. Elster, M.D. (Co-chair)
Naomi J. Kuznets, Ph.D.
Janet E. Gans, Ph.D.
Missy Fleming, Ph.D.
Patricia B. Levenberg, Ph.D.
Katherine H. Voegtle, Ph.D.
Kelly J. Towey
Mary F. Kizer

Special appreciation goes to Janet E. Gans, Ph.D., and Patricia B. Levenberg, Ph.D., who helped write and edit various sections of the book; to Beth Alexander, M.D., who helped write a section on reimbursement; to Kelly Towey for her overall technical assistance; to Robert C. Rinaldi, Ph.D., Director of the AMA's Division of Health Science, for his continued support of the GAPS project; to Lloyd Kolbe, Ph.D., and Mary Vernon, M.D., of the CDC for their vision and advice throughout the development of GAPS; and to many other AMA staff members who helped make this book possible.

Graphics Design (Chicago): Gregory Chambers

The authors wish to express their appreciation to the following people who reviewed chapters for this book:

Vincent A. Fulginiti, M.D.   Anne C. Petersen, Ph.D.
Thomas Houston, M.D.   John Santelli, M.D., M.P.H.
Marc S. Jacobson, M.D.   John Schowalter, M.D.
Michael D. Klitzner, Ph.D.   Mary Story, Ph.D.
Barbara Long, M.D.   Katherine Voegtle, Ph.D.
Donald P. Orr, M.D.   Esther Wender, M.D.

A list of additional people who reviewed material and helped formulate the GAPS recommendations can be found in *Guidelines for Adolescent Preventive Services*, a monograph published by the AMA, Department of Adolescent Health.

Financial support for GAPS was provided through Grant U63-CCU503075-01 from the Division of Adolescent and School Health, National Center for Chronic Disease Prevention and Health Promotion, Centers for Disease Control and Prevention.

Introduction

From a traditional medical perspective, adolescents enjoy a particularly good state of health. Their morbidity rates for certain organic diseases such as heart disease and cancer, which typically afflict adults, are historically low. Likewise, other disorders that may arise during adolescence, such as hypertension and hyperlipidemia, although worrisome, usually cause severe health problems in later life. Adolescence, however, is a time of significant change that can lead to emotional disorders and health-risk behaviors, some of which may cause serious morbidity and mortality. Depression, suicidal ideation, unsafe sexual behaviors, alcohol and drug use, use of tobacco products, and unintentional injuries are just a few of the significant health problems facing adolescents today. These problems are reflected in the following statistics (1–5):

- By age 11, one in five adolescents has smoked cigarettes, and by the age of 15, one in seven adolescents smokes on a daily basis. Overall, two in three high school seniors have tried smoking, and one in three smokes cigarettes regularly.

- By age 11, approximately one in eleven adolescents has had his/her first drink of alcohol, and by their 15th birthday more than one in three adolescents have drunk excessively at least once. Overall, nine out of ten high school seniors have used alcohol, and two in three have drunk excessively.

- By age 15, one in four females and one in three males have had sexual intercourse. By age 18, one in four adolescents will have had a pregnancy, and this number will increase to more than four in ten by age 20. There are over 1 million pregnancies each year in females under the age 20.

- Over one in four adolescents in grades 9–12 have thought seriously about suicide and one in twelve adolescents has actually attempted suicide.

- Over 500,000 adolescents contract gonorrhea each year, and 25% of AIDS cases involve young adults who probably became infected with the human immunodeficiency virus during adolescence.

- Over 50% of adolescent deaths are attributable to injuries from motor vehicle accidents, homicide, and suicide.

Five conclusions can be drawn from adolescent health research of the past decade: (1) the health threats for adolescents today are predominantly behavioral rather than biomedical, (2) more of today's adolescents are involved in health behaviors with the potential for serious consequences, (3) today's adolescents are involved in health-risk behaviors at earlier ages than past generations of adolescents, (4) many, but not all, adolescents engage in multiple health-risk behaviors simultaneously, and (5) most youths engage in some type of personal behavior that threatens their health and well-being.

The reasons for these findings are varied and may include: adverse societal influences, such as unemployment, poverty, and the disintegration of neighborhoods as units of social support; declining availability of parents and other adults to nurture and support adolescents during their development; and greater opportunities for encounters with violence and increased exposure to lethal agents, such as guns or HIV infection. Regardless of the causes, contemporary medicine is faced with a difficult question: how should it respond to the health crisis of today's youth? As medical technologies and therapies have developed in response to new biological threats, so too must preventive strategies be developed and implemented to respond to the challenges threatening the health of adolescents.

Some physicians and health planners, however, may question the role of medicine in behavioral health problems and express concern that the "medicalization" of these problems will only increase health care costs. Others may suspect that expanding clinical preventive services is simply a way for physicians to increase their income. Still others may urge that greater emphasis in medicine be directed at preventing the leading cause of premature death and disability among adults, namely cardiovascular disease. This would require targeting services at children and adolescents to prevent smoking, improve eating habits, promote exercise, and identify and treat early onset of hypertension and hyperlipidemia.

Stimulated by the recommendations for clinical preventive services that were developed by the U.S. Preventive Services Task Force, the Public Health Service's national health objectives for the year 2000, and recent advances in adolescent health research, a growing number of health professionals are advocating the development of clinical strategies aimed at improving adolescent health and well-being through primary and secondary prevention efforts. Care must be exercised to ensure this strategy is pragmatic and reasonable, has a relatively good chance to be effective, and has either no risk or low risk of causing harm to adolescents or their parents.

Guidelines for Adolescent Preventive Services (GAPS) is a clinical strategy that meets these criteria. GAPS recommends that, in addition to treating physical disease and the medical consequences of adolescent health-risk behaviors, physicians should also actively attempt to prevent or modify these behaviors. This strategy is predicated not only on concern for the long-term health outcomes of lifestyles and health behaviors that begin during adolescence, but also on concern for the immediate health and well-being of adolescents. GAPS represents an ambitious strategy. For it to succeed, physicians and other health professionals, adolescents, and parents will need to work in partnership toward a common goal.

Improving adolescent health will be challenging because it requires a broad prevention strategy encompassing many aspects of community life. Schools have responded to this challenge through the expansion of health education curricula and implementation of special prevention programs. Likewise, many youth-serving organizations and churches have responded by implementing health promotion programs for adolescents and families. Cities and government agencies have responded with public information campaigns and passage of health regulations directed at protecting the safety of adolescents. GAPS provides a strategy for how physicians and other primary health providers can also address the challenge of improving adolescent health.

WHAT IS GAPS?

Guidelines for Adolescent Preventive Services (GAPS) is a comprehensive package of recommendations for primary care physicians and other health providers who see adolescent patients in clinical settings. These recommendations are designed to be delivered during a series of annual preventive service health visits between the ages of 11 and 21.

GAPS provide a framework for the organization and content of routine health care for adolescents. Some GAPS recommendations are already performed on a routine basis by many physicians. For example, 58–72% of physicians screen children with a family history of cardiovascular disease for elevated cholesterol levels (6–8). In a national survey, Nader and associates found that most physicians reported that they measure adolescents for blood pressure and that they routinely counsel adolescents about diet, exercise, and smoking (6). For many adolescents, GAPS would not necessitate an additional clinic visit. Many adolescents already see a physician at least once a year for routine health examinations to meet athletic, camp, or school requirements.

However, physicians do not currently deliver a comprehensive range of clinical preventive services to adolescents on a systematic basis. Barriers to clinical preventive services include uncertainties about what services to provide, how to manage identified problems, and the effectiveness of preventive services (8, 9). For example, a majority of physicians apparently believe that screening children for risk of cardiovascular disease is necessary. Although a majority perform screening procedures, only 20–30% of physicians believe they can be effective in helping children reduce their risk of subsequent disease (6–8). GAPS addresses these barriers by presenting concise recommendations based on available scientific research and expert opinion. GAPS offers primary care providers a well-delineated package of clinical preventive services that are practical to implement, that address the conditions posing the greatest burden of suffering to adolescents, and that are likely to be effective. Although best implemented as a comprehensive package of services, the emphasis on individual recommendations during a particular visit will vary depending on the age, health-risk status, and health care needs of the adolescent, and on the social circumstances of the adolescent's family.

GAPS recommendations are directed at improving health through the use of primary and secondary preventive interventions, such as health guidance, immunizations, and early detection and treatment.

GAPS does not address tertiary, or therapeutic, interventions; nor does it address interventions directed at either acute or chronic medical management. Guides for managing these types of health problems are contained in a variety of textbooks and scientific journals on adolescent medicine. The target population for GAPS, therefore, is adolescents who appear relatively healthy and do not already have diagnosed conditions that are targeted by GAPS screening recommendations. Although some clinical adaptation may be necessary, adolescents with chronic health conditions or disabilities should be provided with GAPS services as well.

The impetus for developing GAPS was the belief that the continued decline in adolescent health indicators over the past decade necessitated a fundamental change in the delivery of adolescent health services.

The clinical visit provides an opportunity for health promotion and disease prevention, which is currently underutilized. During this visit, physicians will be able to provide health guidance to both adolescents and their parents. The term "health guidance," as used in GAPS, encompasses health education, health counseling, and anticipatory guidance. Annual health visits also provide physicians the opportunity to identify adolescents who have recently initiated health-risk behaviors or who have early stages of physical or emotional disorders.

Research suggests that efforts to promote healthy behaviors are most effective when adolescents receive consistent health messages that are reinforced by creditable sources from different settings (10). The package of GAPS preventive services is designed to complement and reinforce the health education provided by schools, parents, and other community groups.

Effective implementation of GAPS recommendations will necessitate involvement of support staff, as well as the development of a practice environment supportive of health promotion. By organizing their practice to provide comprehensive preventive services, physicians will make an important contribution to improving the health and well-being of adolescents.

The GAPS package contains 24 recommendations in four types, directed at 14 separate health topics. A full list of the recommendations follows this Introduction. In summary:

- Three recommendations address the system of health care delivery.

- Seven recommendations focus on the use of health guidance to promote the health and well-being of adolescents and their families.

- Thirteen recommendations promote the use of screening to identify conditions relatively common to adolescents that cause significant suffering either during adolescence or later in life.

- One recommendation proposes the use of immunizations for the primary prevention of selected infectious diseases.

The fourteen health topics include:

- Parenting and family adjustment

- Psychosocial adjustment

- Intentional and unintentional injuries

- Dietary habits, eating disorders, and obesity

- Physical fitness

- Sexual behavior, STDs, and unintended pregnancy

- Hypertension

- Hyperlipidemia

- Use of tobacco products

- Use of alcohol, other drugs, and anabolic steroids

- Severe or recurrent depression and suicide

- Physical, sexual, and emotional abuse

- Learning and school problems

- Infectious diseases

For some health topics, the preventive strategy includes a recommendation for either health guidance, screening, or immunization services. Other health topics, however, are addressed by a combination of services. Table I.1 shows the relation between health topics and type of recommendation.

WHAT ARE PRACTICE GUIDELINES AND WHY ARE THEY NECESSARY?

In response to expansion of medical technology and concern for rising medical costs, increased attention has been directed by the private and public health care sectors at defining parameters for clinical care. These parameters have various names, including practice parameters and practice guidelines. As defined by the Institute of Medicine (IOM):

> Practice guidelines are a systematically developed set of statements(s) to assist health professionals with patient decisions about appropriate health care for specific clinical circumstances (11).

Imbedded in this definition are several terms that indicate the shift in how patient care recommendations are developed.

The IOM definition states that practice guidelines are a "systematically developed" set of statements. The term "systematic" implies an orderly process of development and not one in which recommendations merely evolve from current standards of medical practice. Practice guidelines developed systematically target specific conditions, actions, or goals. Recommenda-

Table I.1. Associations Among the Three Types of GAPS Recommendations (R) and the Fourteen Health Topics

Health Topics	Type of Recommendation		
	Health Guidance	Screening	Immunizations
Parenting and Family Adjustment	R4		
Psychosocial Adjustment	R5		
Intentional and Unintentional Injury	R4, R6		
Dietary Habits, Eating Disorders, and Obesity	R7	R13	
Physical Fitness	R8		
Sexual Development and the Adverse Consequences of Sexual Intercourse	R9	R16-R19	R24
Hypertension		R11	
Hyperlipidemia		R12	
Use of Tobacco Products	R10	R14	
Use of Alcohol, Other Drugs, and Anabolic Steroids	R10	R15	
Severe or Recurrent Depression and Suicide		R20	
Physical, Sexual and Emotional Abuse		R21	
Learning and School Problems		R22	
Infectious Diseases		R23	R24

tions that evolve from community practices generally lack specificity regarding intended outcomes. Practice guidelines are now commonly developed by one of two systematic approaches (9, 11).

With one approach, recommendations are based upon opinions of national experts. Information used in this approach includes an orderly review of current professional opinion, the health needs of the targeted population, and data from nonexperimentally designed research. While the results of the research literature are considered, recommendations developed by "expert opinion" are not bound by the availability of existing scientific studies. The recommendations developed by expert opinion may be conceptually sound, but they do not necessarily reflect conclusions drawn from scientific evidence.

With the second method of guideline development, recommendations are based on analyses of studies demonstrating the efficacy of a particular intervention in controlled clinical trials. This approach is most appropriate when evaluating the efficacy of procedures that have immediate and easily measurable outcomes, such as laboratory tests and therapeutic regimens. However, evaluating health guidance and behavioral screening recommendations present different challenges that are not as well addressed by outcomes based on research. For example, physician intervention will be but one factor influencing adolescent behavior; various outcomes, such as emotional well-being and improved lifestyles, are difficult to quantify and measure; and the effect of some interventions on health outcomes might not be noted for decades. In addition, the efficacy of some preventive interventions, such as screening for sexual behavior or alcohol use, are not applicable to a clinical trial because it would be unethical to screen some adolescents for health-risk behaviors and not screen others.

Another term used in the IOM definition, "practice guidelines," connotes flexibility in the application of the set of recommendations. Depending on the certainty of the effectiveness of the proposed intervention, recommendations can be viewed as standards or criteria, guidelines, or suggestions or options (11, 12). Practically, the difference among these three types of recommendations is the rigidity by which the policy is advocated—the greater the certainty of the outcome, the stronger or more rigid the policy recommendation. Care must be taken, however, not to always interpret the lack of certainty for an outcome as a negative finding. The lack of certainty regarding the effectiveness of many GAPS recommendations, for example, results primarily from a scarcity of studies done on adolescent clinical preventive services, and not from studies of interventions that suggest no effect.

The implementation of systematic practice guidelines can have various beneficial results. These include reducing clinically significant variation in the delivery of services and procedures by improving clinical practice, reducing clinically significant variations in health outcomes, and reducing the long-term cost of health care (9). Practice guidelines also provide physicians with education about the most critical health issues affecting the targeted population.

Prior to implementing practice guidelines, consideration should also be given to the potential for adverse outcomes and to ensuring that the preventive intervention has the probability of causing more good than harm. Examples of untoward outcomes include an increase in the short-term cost of health care (i.e., costs of additional clinical visits, screening procedures, therapeutic interventions), mislabeling of vulnerability, patient anxiety produced by the identification of a false-positive result, and a reduction of the office time given to other, possibly more effective, interventions.

HOW WERE GAPS RECOMMENDATIONS DEVELOPED?

GAPS recommendations were developed by the American Medical Association with the assistance of a national scientific advisory board. This group consisted of experts in medicine (including adolescent medicine, child and adolescent psychiatry, obstetrics and gynecology, internal medicine, and family practice), social and behavioral science (including health psychology, developmental psychology, health education, public health research), and health insurance.

The methodology used to develop GAPS recommendations followed criteria similar to protocol established by the American Medical Association and by the Institute of Medicine (11, 13). These criteria addressed the following:

1. Validity: If the guidelines are followed, they should lead to the expected outcome.
2. Reliability: Other people, if given the same evidence, would identify the same recommendations.
3. Clinical applicability: Guidelines should clearly define the target population.
4. Clinical flexibility: Guidelines should identify the expected exceptions to the recommendations and how they may be used in different clinical settings.

As new information becomes evident, GAPS recommendations will need to be updated.

WHAT ARE THE UNIQUE ASPECTS OF GAPS RECOMMENDATIONS?

GAPS provides, for the first time, national systematically developed recommendations for delivering a package of adolescent clinical preventive services. While sets of recommendations exist for screening or immunizations related to single medical issues, there is no comprehensive set of guidelines that address the contemporary health problems experienced by youth.

An additional, unique aspect of GAPS is the recommendation for annual preventive service visits. Historically, regularly scheduled well-child prevention visits were limited to infants and toddlers. The GAPS national scientific advisory board concluded that the current state of adolescent health necessitates a fundamental change in the way preventive services are delivered. The new strategy recommends annual preventive service visits that focus on health guidance, immunizations, and screening for physical, emotional, and behavioral conditions.

A final unique aspect of GAPS is that it includes recommendations for health guidance for families of adolescents. This approach represents a change from previous intervention strategies that focus predominantly on adolescents. The GAPS national scientific advisory board considered that parents need guidance to help them meet the changing physical and emotional needs of their adolescent.

Table I.2 summarizes how GAPS recommendations differ from traditional medical practice for adolescents.

WHAT IS THE ANTICIPATED IMPACT OF GAPS SERVICES?

GAPS recommendations will contribute to a community strategy that promotes the general health and well-being of adolescents and prevents serious morbidity and mortality. The health problems addressed by GAPS have an enormous financial impact on society. For example, the total direct medical expense associated with adolescent pregnancy, treatment of STD infections (HIV infection and AIDS), alcohol and drug treatment, motor vehicle accidents, and mental health treatment is approximately $30 billion per year. This preliminary figure was calculated by multiplying the number of adolescents with each health condition by an average 1992 cost for managing that condition. The estimate is conservative—it does not include long-term

Table I.2. How GAPS Differs from the Traditional Practice of Medical Care for Adolescents

GAPS Recommendations	Traditional Medical Care
Preventive interventions provided by the physician complement health education that adolescents receive in their family, school, and community.	Physician role is generally considered independent of health education offered by family, schools, and the community.
Emphasis is on health promotion as well as disease prevention.	Diagnostic and therapeutic interventions are disease-oriented.
Preventive interventions target "social morbidities", such as alcohol and other drug use, suicide, STDs (including HIV), unintended pregnancy, and eating disorders.	Emphasis is on biomedical problems, including the medical consequences of health risk behaviors, such as STDs and pregnancy.
Emphasis is on screening for "co-morbidities," i.e., adolescent participation in clusters of specific health risk behaviors.	Emphasis is on the diagnosis and treatment of categorical health conditions.
Annual visits allow early detection of health problems and provide an opportunity for health guidance, immunizations, and the development of a therapeutic relationship.	Visits scheduled as needed for acute care episodes, follow-up care, management of chronic conditions, or sports examinations.
Comprehensive physical examinations are performed once during early, once during middle, and once during late adolescence.	Current standards vary from no recommendation on periodicity, to examinations every two years during adolescence, to examinations required for participation in sports.
Parents receive health guidance at least twice during their child's adolescence.	The nature, type, and frequency of health guidance is left to the discretion of the physician.

costs of medical management, entitlement programs, or lost wages associated with disabilities, chronic health problems, or adolescent child bearing. Also excluded are the long-term costs of behaviors that begin during adolescence, such as smoking and physical inactivity, but do not cause morbidity until later in life. Thus, unless current preventive strategies change, adolescent morbidities will continue to result in a substantial economic cost to society, in addition to the widespread and immeasurable cost in human suffering.

The effectiveness of GAPS recommendations in promoting health and preventing disease depends on two major factors: (1) the ability of physicians to implement the recommendations and (2) the likelihood that the interventions, if performed properly, will promote healthy lifestyles or will lead to an early diagnosis that can shorten the course of a clinical disorder or change behavior. Until GAPS is used on a widespread and systematic basis, the impact of the recommendations will not be known. Like many health issues that affect large numbers of people, however, relatively modest rates of success in behavioral change can have profound effects when viewed in perspective with the entire population.

The projected cost of GAPS services can be calculated by multiplying the estimated costs of periodic services (i.e., cholesterol screening, Pap test, etc.) and adding this amount to the estimated costs of annual clinic visits. Based upon an estimated 30 minutes per GAPS visit, and a youth population of 39 million between the ages of 11 and 21, preliminary estimates are that GAPS will cost approximately $9 billion per year to implement fully. A major portion of this figure, about 30%, is for the cost of the annual health visit. Because many adolescents each year already have a general examination for camp, school, or athletics, a sizeable amount of these costs do not entail new financial expenditures. They are already incurred by families or by insurers. GAPS recommendations for laboratory tests (i.e., such as cholesterol screening and STD testing) and immunizations also represent existing costs.

HOW THE BOOK IS ORGANIZED

This book is intended to describe how the GAPS recommendations were developed and the scientific justification for these recommendations. A discussion of important aspects of the preventive service visit is also included. *AMA Guidelines for Adolescent Preventive Services* predominantly contains information related to practice policy; materials to help physicians implement GAPS recommendations will be available from the AMA at a future date.

Chapter 1 addresses the rationale for the recommendations pertaining to the delivery of health services. Chapters 2–5 address the rationale for health guidance recommendations, while Chapters 6–14 address the rationale for health topics with screening recommendations. Chapter 15 addresses the rationale for the recommendation concerning immunizations. Most chapters include a summary of the recommended *Prevention Strategy*, a *Discussion* that provides background information and *Justifies* the recommendation, and a brief discussion of *Clinical Application/Intervention*. The justification section is organized by questions that cover critical aspects of the scientific linkage between screening and outcome. Finally, Chapter 16 describes components of the preventive service visit, including a chart outlining recommended services for each visit from ages 11 to 21.

REFERENCES

1. Blum R. Contemporary threats to adolescent health in the United States. JAMA 1987;257:3390–3395.
2. Gans JE, Blyth DA, Elster AB, Lundgren L. America's Adolescents: How Healthy Are They? Chicago: American Medical Association, 1990.
3. Bachman JG, Johnston LD, O'Malley PM. Monitoring the Future: Questionnaire Responses From the Nation's High School Seniors 1988. Ann Arbor, MI: Institute for Social Research, 1991.
4. The Alan Guttmacher Institute. Facts in Brief: Teenage Sexual and Reproductive Behavior. New York: The Alan Guttmacher Institute, 1992.
5. Centers for Disease Control. Attempted suicide among high school students— United States, 1990. MMWR 1991;40:633–635.
6. Nader PR, Taras HL, Sallis JF, Patterson TL. Adult heart disease prevention in childhood: a national survey of pediatricians' practices and attitudes. Pediatrics 1987; 79:843–850.
7. Kimm SYS, Payne GH, Lakatos E, Darby C, Sparrow A. Management of cardiovascular disease risk factors in children. Am J Dis Child 1990;144:967–972.
8. Arneson T, Luepker R, Ririe P, Sinaiko A. Cholesterol screening by primary care pediatricians. A study of attitudes and practices in the Minneapolis-St. Paul metropolitan area. Pediatrics 1992;89:502–505.
9. US Preventive Services Task Force. Guide to Clinical Preventive Services: An Assessment of the Effectiveness of 169 Interventions. Baltimore: Williams & Wilkins, 1989.
10. Elster A, Panzarine S, Holt K, eds. AMA State of the Art Conference on Adolescent Health Promotion: Proceedings. Rockville, MD: National Clearinghouse on Maternal and Child Health, 1993.
11. Field MJ, Lohr KN. Clinical Practice Guidelines: Directions for a New Program. Washington, DC: National Academy Press, 1990.

12. Eddy DM. Designing a practice policy: standards, guidelines, and options. JAMA 1990;263:3077–3084.
13. AMA Practice Parameters Partnership. Attributes to Guide the Development of Practice Parameters. Chicago: American Medical Association, 1990.
14. Cromer BA, McLean CS, Health FP. A critical review of comprehensive health screening in adolescents. J Adolesc Health 1992;13:1S–65S.
15. Himes JH, Dietz WH. Guidelines for overweight in adolescent preventive services: recommendations from the Expert Committee on Clinical Guidelines for Overweight in Adolescent Preventive Services (in preparation).

Guidelines for Adolescent Preventive Services

I. RECOMMENDATIONS FOR DELIVERY OF HEALTH SERVICES

Recommendation 1: From ages 11 to 21, all adolescents should have an annual routine health visit.

- These visits should address the biomedical and psychosocial aspects of health, and they should focus on preventive services.
- Adolescents should have a complete physical examination during three of these preventive service visits. One should be performed during early adolescence (age 11–14), one during middle adolescence (age 15–17) and one during late adolescence (age 18–21), unless more frequent examinations are warranted by clinical signs or symptoms.

Recommendation 2: Preventive services should be age and developmentally appropriate, and they should be sensitive to individual and sociocultural differences.

Recommendation 3: Physicians should establish office policies regarding confidential care for adolescents and how parents will be involved in that care. These policies should be made clear to adolescents and their parents.

II. RECOMMENDATIONS FOR HEALTH GUIDANCE

Recommendation 4: Parents or other adult caregivers of adolescents should receive health guidance at least once during early adolescence, once during middle adolescence and, preferably, once during late adolescence.

This includes providing information about:

- Normative adolescent development, including information about physical, sexual, and emotional development.

- Signs and symptoms of disease and emotional distress.

- Parenting behaviors that promote healthy adolescent adjustment.

- Benefits parents can realize by discussing health-related behaviors with their adolescent, planning family activities, and acting as role models for health-related behaviors.

- Methods for helping their adolescent avoid potentially harmful behaviors, such as:

Monitoring and managing the adolescent's use of motor vehicles, especially if he or she is a new driver.

Avoiding having weapons in the home. Parents who have weapons in the home should be advised to make them inaccessible to adolescents. If adolescents have weapons, parents and other adult caregivers should ensure that adolescents follow weapon safety procedures.

Removing weapons and potentially lethal medications from the homes of adolescents who have suicidal intent.

Monitoring their adolescent's social and recreational activities to restrict sexual behavior and use of tobacco, alcohol, and other drugs.

Recommendation 5: All adolescents should receive health guidance annually to promote a better understanding of their physical growth, psychosocial and psychosexual development, and the importance of becoming actively involved in decisions regarding their health care.

Recommendation 6: All adolescents should receive health guidance annually to promote the reduction of injuries.

Health guidance for injury prevention includes:

- Counseling to avoid the use of alcohol or other substances while using motor or recreational vehicles, or where impaired judgment may lead to injury.

- Counseling to use safety devices, including seat belts, motorcycle and bicycle helmets, and appropriate athletic protective devices.

- Counseling to resolve interpersonal conflicts without violence.

- Counseling to avoid the use of weapons and/or promote weapon safety.

- Counseling to promote appropriate physical conditioning before exercise.

Recommendation 7: All adolescents should receive health guidance annually about dietary habits, including the benefits of a healthy diet and ways to achieve a healthy diet and safe weight management.

Recommendation 8: All adolescents should receive health guidance annually about the benefits of exercise and should be encouraged to engage in safe exercise on a regular basis.

Recommendation 9: All adolescents should receive health guidance annually regarding responsible sexual behaviors, including abstinence. Latex condoms to prevent STDs (including HIV infection) and appropriate methods of birth control should be made available with instructions on how to use them effectively.
Health guidance for sexual responsibility includes:

- Counseling that abstinence from sexual intercourse is the most effective way to prevent pregnancy and sexually transmissible diseases (STDs), including HIV infection.

- Counseling on how human immunodeficiency virus (HIV) is transmitted, on the dangers of the disease, and on the effectiveness of latex condoms in preventing STDs, including HIV infection.

- Counseling to reinforce responsible sexual behavior in adolescents who are not currently sexually active and in those who are using birth control and condoms appropriately.

- Counseling on the need for adolescents to protect themselves and their partners from pregnancy, STDs (including HIV infection), and sexual exploitation.

Recommendation 10: All adolescents should receive health guidance annually to promote avoidance of tobacco, alcohol and abusable substances, and anabolic steroids.

III. RECOMMENDATIONS FOR SCREENING

Recommendation 11: All adolescents should be screened annually for hypertension according to the protocol developed by the National Heart, Lung, and Blood Institute Second Task Force on Blood Pressure Control in Children.

- Adolescents with either systolic or diastolic pressures at or above the 90th percentile for gender and age should have blood pressure (BP) measurements repeated at three different times within one month, under similar physical conditions, to confirm baseline values.

- Adolescents with baseline BP values greater than the 95th percentile for gender and age should have a complete biomedical evaluation to establish treatment options. Adolescents with BP values between the 90th and 95th percentile should be assessed for obesity and their blood pressure monitored every six months.

Recommendation 12: Selected adolescents should be screened to determine their risk of developing hyperlipidemia and adult coronary heart disease, following the protocol developed by the Expert Panel on Blood Cholesterol Levels in Children and Adolescents.

- Adolescents whose parents have a serum cholesterol level greater than 240 mg/dl and adolescents who are over 19 years of age should be screened for a total blood cholesterol level (nonfasting) at least once.

- Adolescents with an unknown family history or who have multiple risk factors for future cardiovascular disease (e.g., smoking, hypertension, obesity, diabetes mellitus, excessive consumption of dietary saturated fats and cholesterol) may be screened for total serum cholesterol level (nonfasting) at least once at the discretion of the physician.

- Adolescents with blood cholesterol values less than 170 mg/dl should have the test repeated within five years. Those with values between 170 and 199 mg/dl should have a repeated test. If the average of the two tests is below 170 mg/dl, total blood cholesterol level should be reassessed within five years. A lipoprotein analysis should be done if the average cholesterol value from the two tests is 170 mg/dl or higher, or if the result of the initial test was 200 mg/dl or greater.

- Adolescents who have a parent or grandparent with coronary artery disease, peripheral vascular disease, cerebrovascular disease, or sudden cardiac death at age 55 or younger should be screened with a fasting lipoprotein analysis.

- Treatment options are based on the average of two assessments of low-density lipoprotein cholesterol. Values below 110 mg/dl are acceptable; values between 110 and 129 mg/dl are borderline. The lipoprotein status should be re-evaluated in one year. Adolescents with values of 130 mg/dl or greater should be referred for further medical evaluation and treatment.

Recommendation 13: All adolescents should be screened annually for eating disorders and obesity by determining weight and stature, and asking about body image and dieting patterns.

- Adolescents should be assessed for organic disease, anorexia nervosa, or bulimia if any of the following are found:
  - Weight loss greater than 10% of previous weight
  - Recurrent dieting when not overweight
  - Use of self-induced emesis, laxatives, starvation, or diuretics to lose weight
  - Distorted body image
  - Body mass index (weight/height^2) below the fifth percentile

- Adolescents with a body mass index (BMI) equal to or greater than the 95th percentile for age and gender are considered overweight and should have a more in-depth dietary and health assessment to determine psychosocial morbidity and risk for future cardiovascular disease.

- Adolescents with a BMI between the 85th and 94th percentile are at risk for becoming overweight. A dietary and health assessment to determine psychosocial morbidity and risk for future cardiovascular disease should be performed on such youths if any one of the following is identified:
  - their BMI has increased by two or more units during the previous 12 months;
  - there is a family history of premature heart disease, obesity, hypertension, or diabetes mellitus;
  - they express concern about their weight;
  - they have elevated serum cholesterol levels or blood pressure.

  If this assessment is negative, these adolescents should be provided general dietary and exercise counseling and monitored annually.

Recommendation 14: All adolescents should be asked annually about their use of tobacco products, including cigarettes and smokeless tobacco.

- Adolescents who use tobacco products should be assessed further to determine their pattern of use.

- A cessation plan should be provided for adolescents who use tobacco products.

Recommendation 15: All adolescents should be asked annually about their use of alcohol and other abusable substances, and about their use of over-the-counter or prescription drugs for nonmedical purposes, including anabolic steroids.

- Adolescents who report any use of alcohol or other drugs or inappropriate use of medicines during the past year should be assessed further regarding family history; circumstances surrounding use; amount and frequency of use; attitudes and motivation about use; use of other drugs; and the adequacy of physical, psychosocial, and school functioning.

- Adolescents whose substance use endangers their health should be referred for counseling and mental health treatment, as appropriate.

- Adolescents who use anabolic steroids should be counseled to stop.

- Use of urine toxicology for the routine screening of adolescents is not recommended.

- Adolescents who use alcohol or other drugs should also be asked about their sexual behavior and their use of tobacco products.

Recommendation 16: All adolescents should be asked annually about involvement in sexual behaviors that may result in unintended pregnancy and STDs, including HIV infection.

- Sexually active adolescents should be asked about their use and motivation to use condoms and contraceptive methods, their sexual orientation, the number of sexual partners they have had in the past six months, if they have exchanged sex for money or drugs, and their history of prior pregnancy or STDs.

- Adolescents at risk for pregnancy, STDs (including HIV), or sexual exploitation should be counseled on how to reduce this risk.

- Sexually active adolescents should also be asked about their use of tobacco products, alcohol, and other drugs.

Recommendation 17: Sexually active adolescents should be screened for STDs.

- STD screening includes:
  - a cervical culture (females) or urine leukocyte esterase analysis (males) to screen for gonorrhea;
  - an immunologic test of cervical fluid (female) or urine leukocyte esterase analysis (male) to screen for genital chlamydia;
  - a serologic test for syphilis if they have lived in an area endemic for syphilis, have had other STDs, have had more than one sexual partner within the last six months, have exchanged sex for drugs or money, or are males who have engaged in sex with other males;
  - an evaluation for human papilloma virus by visual inspection (males and females) and by Pap test (females).

- If a presumptive test for STDs is positive, tests to make a definitive diagnosis should be performed, a treatment plan should be instituted according to guidelines developed by the Centers for Disease Control and Prevention, and the use of condoms should be encouraged.

- The frequency of screening for STDs depends on the sexual practices of the individual and the history of previous STDs.

Recommendation 18: Adolescents at risk for HIV infection should be offered confidential HIV screening with the ELISA and confirmatory test.

- Risk status includes having used intravenous drugs, having had other STD infections, having lived in an area with a high prevalence of STDs and HIV infection, having had more than one sexual partner in the last six months, having exchanged sex for drugs or money, being male and having engaged in sex with other males, or having had a sexual partner who is at risk for HIV infection.

- Testing should be performed only after informed consent is obtained from the adolescent.

- Testing should be performed only in conjunction with pretest and posttest counseling.

- The frequency of screening for HIV infection should be determined by the risk factors of the individual.

Recommendation 19: Female adolescents who are sexually active or any female 18 or older should be screened annually for cervical cancer by use of a Pap test.

Adolescents with a positive Pap test should be referred for further diagnostic assessment and management.

Recommendation 20: All adolescents should be asked annually about behaviors or emotions that indicate recurrent or severe depression or risk of suicide.

- Screening for depression or suicidal risk should be performed on adolescents who exhibit cumulative risk as determined by declining school grades, chronic melancholy, family dysfunction, homosexual orientation, history of physical or sexual abuse, alcohol or other drug use, previous suicide attempt, and suicidal plans.

- If suicidal risk is suspected, adolescents should be evaluated immediately. They should be referred to a psychiatrist or other mental health professional, or they should be hospitalized.

- Nonsuicidal adolescents with symptoms of severe or recurrent depression should be referred to a psychiatrist or other mental health professional for treatment.

Recommendation 21: All adolescents should be asked annually about a history of emotional, physical, and sexual abuse.

- If abuse is suspected, adolescents should be assessed to determine the circumstances surrounding abuse and the presence of physical, emotional, and psychosocial consequences, including involvement in health-risk behaviors.

- Health providers should be aware of local laws about the reporting of abuse to appropriate state officials, in addition to ethical and legal issues regarding how to protect the confidentiality of the adolescent patient.

- Adolescents who report emotional or psychosocial sequelae should be referred to a psychiatrist or other mental health professional for evaluation and treatment.

Recommendation 22: All adolescents should be asked annually about learning or school problems.

- Adolescents who report a history of truancy, repeated absences, or poor or declining performance should be assessed for the presence of conditions that could interfere with school success. These include learning disability, attention-deficit hyperactivity disorder, medical problems, sexual abuse, family dysfunction, mental disorders, or alcohol or other drug use.

- This assessment, and the subsequent management plan, should be coordinated with school personnel and with the adolescent's parents or caregivers.

Recommendation 23: Adolescents should receive a tuberculin skin test if they have been exposed to active tuberculosis, have lived in a homeless shelter, have been incarcerated, have lived in or come from an area with a high prevalence of tuberculosis, or currently work in a health care setting.

- Adolescents with a positive tuberculin test should be treated according to treatment guidelines developed by the Centers for Disease Control and Prevention.

- The frequency of testing depends on risk factors of the individual adolescent.

IV. RECOMMENDATIONS FOR IMMUNIZATIONS

Recommendation 24: All adolescents should receive prophylactic immunizations according to the guidelines established by the federally convened Advisory Committee on Immunization Practices.

- Adolescents should receive a bivalent Td vaccine 10 years after their previous DPT vaccination.

- All adolescents should receive a second trivalent MMR vaccination, unless there is documentation of two vaccinations earlier during childhood. An MMR should not be given to adolescents who are pregnant.

- Susceptible adolescents who engage in high-risk behaviors should be vaccinated against hepatitis B virus. This includes adolescents who have had more than one sexual partner during the previous six months, have exchanged sex for drugs or money, are males who have engaged in sex with other males, or have used intravenous drugs. Widespread use of the hepatitis B vaccine is encouraged because risk factors are often not easily identifiable among adolescents. Universal hepatitis B vaccination should be implemented in communities where intravenous drug use, adolescent pregnancy, and/or STD infections are common.

CHAPTER 1

Rationale and Recommendations: Delivery of Health Services to Adolescents

PREVENTION STRATEGY

GAPS recommends that all adolescents have an annual preventive service visit from the ages of 11 to 21. These visits should address physical and psychosocial aspects of health, and they should focus on promoting healthy lifestyles as well as preventing disease. Unless more frequent examinations are warranted by clinical signs or symptoms, these visits should include three complete physical examinations: one during early adolescence (11–14), one during middle adolescence (15–17) and one during late adolescence (18–21). The GAPS national scientific advisory board chose to focus on young people from ages 11 to 21 to ensure services are provided to youths from the beginning to the end of adolescence. The guideline for annual preventive service visits is addressed by GAPS Recommendation 1.

To be effective, these preventive service visits should be appropriate to age and development, and they should take into account individual cultural differences. Physicians and health providers will need to emphasize components of the preventive service visit differently, depending on individual patient and family characteristics. This guideline is addressed by GAPS Recommendation 2.

Finally, GAPS recommends providers establish office policies regarding confidential care for adolescents, and how parents will be involved. This policy should be made clear to adolescents and their families. The need for confidential health services is addressed by GAPS Recommendation 3.

1

ANNUAL PREVENTIVE SERVICE VISITS

JUSTIFICATION

Within the last several decades, adolescent morbidity and mortality have changed dramatically. Physical diseases are no longer the primary cause of death and disability for adolescents (1, 2). Instead, the major health problems of adolescence result from personal behavior, such as intentional and unintentional injury, alcohol and drug use, eating disorders, and sexual behavior that leads to unintended pregnancy and STDs, including HIV infection. In contrast to previous decades, most health problems of contemporary adolescents are preventable.

The adolescent morbidities and mortalities listed above result mostly from health-risk behaviors—behaviors that begin and increase dramatically during early adolescence. The need to initiate prevention efforts with young adolescents is demonstrated in Figure 1.1.

Figure 1.1 shows the number of adolescents at each year of age who (1) experiment with tobacco, alcohol, and drugs for the first time and (2) engage in sexual intercourse for the first time (3, 4). The first use of cigarettes increases during early adolescence, and then declines. The first use of alcohol and marijuana increases somewhat later and also declines later. An increase in first sexual intercourse occurs still later and continues to increase through middle to late adolescence. The figure does not show that the initiation of more serious health-risk behaviors follows similar trends. Consequently, most adolescents who smoke daily, use marijuana daily, and/or drink excessively (e.g., report having been drunk) initiate these behaviors between the ages of 11 and 14.

Three conclusions can be drawn from these data: (1) a substantial number of adolescents initiate experimentation and many begin more serious health-risk behaviors at young ages, (2) screening for health-risk behaviors cannot be limited to any one year of life or any group of adolescents because the age at first involvement varies with the individual and the type of behavior, and (3) many adolescents who have just begun or plan to begin health-risk behaviors will be missed unless they are screened each year.

The justification for annual visits is based on the premise that screening adolescents at regular yearly intervals is necessary to identify those who have recently begun, or are considering, health-risk behaviors; those in whom such behavior has recently escalated to a more serious level; and those who have early onset of emotional or physical disorders. Early identification and intervention may prevent serious health consequences, such as alcohol-related injuries and deaths, attempted suicide, unintended pregnancy, compli-

Figure 1.1. Age at First Involvement in Selected Health-Risk Behaviors

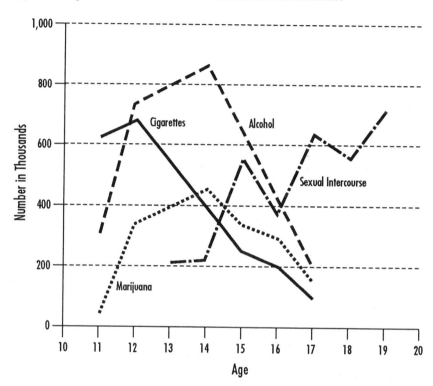

Sources: 1. Bachman J.G., Johnston L.D., O'Malley P.M. Monitoring the Future, 1988. Ann Arbor, MI: Institute for Social Research, 1991. 2. Facts In Brief: Teenage Sexual and Reproductive Behavior. New York: Alan Guttmacher Institute, 1991.

cations from STDs, and transmission of sexually transmitted diseases to other partners. An example of the need for, and potential benefit from, regular screening for sexual activity (with clinical intervention) is that half of all premarital adolescent pregnancies occur within the first six months of initiation of sexual intercourse (5). Forty-two percent of females 15 years of age, 35% of females age 15 to 17, and 15% of 18–19-year-old adolescents postpone contraception more than one year from the time of first intercourse (6, 7). Annual health visits will provide an opportunity to identify adolescents who have recently become sexually active and to provide these youths with appropriate preventive interventions.

In addition to screening for physical, emotional, and behavioral health problems, regular preventive service visits also provide physicians the chance to counsel adolescents and their parents on how to promote healthy life-styles, cope with the physical and emotional stresses of adolescence, and prevent injury. This health guidance can supplement and reinforce information already learned in school and from parents.

Frequent annual visits that focus on health guidance and screening are a departure from the manner in which adolescent health services are currently structured. The question arises as to whether all adolescents need to be seen annually. This question implies that some adolescents are less likely to need yearly clinical preventive services and can be seen less frequently. Most adolescents who experiment with health-risk behaviors, however, are well-adjusted emotionally and do not have characteristics that distinguish them from adolescents who postpone involvement. Because of the range of potential problems, no one measure can accurately predict which youths are at risk for health-threatening behaviors or emotional disorders. For example, adolescents who live in poverty might be more at risk for certain health problems, while adolescents who live in wealth are at risk for others. Demographic characteristics such as family income, family composition, or racial and ethnic background, when used alone, predict some but not all adolescent health problems (1). Because of this argument, the GAPS Scientific Advisory Board recommended a universal rather than targeted strategy for screening and health guidance.

The use of a routine physical examination to detect organic disease among adolescents has a low yield of positive results. In a study done in the early 1970s, Grant and associates found that only 13% of students between the ages of 5 and 18 had a significant abnormality undetected previously (8). Of these, fewer than 30% were identified through physical examination. Physical disorders beginning during adolescence are usually associated with signs and symptoms that can be detected through measurements of height, weight, and blood pressure; or through a brief interim health history, rather than a physical examination. For example, diabetes mellitus, thyroid disorder, and inflammatory bowel disease are often associated with changes in weight, stunted growth, emotional lability, or chronic somatic pain. It is for this reason that GAPS recommends, unless otherwise indicated, a complete physical examination for adolescents every two to three years; that is, once during each stage of adolescence—early, middle, and late.

INDIVIDUALIZED SERVICES

JUSTIFICATION

Although all adolescents experience rapid physical and emotional changes, the trajectory and context of these changes vary widely among individuals. The complexities of adolescent development and the strong influence that culture, ethnicity and race, and poverty have on behavior require that physicians take into account these individual differences to provide effective preventive intervention services.

Physical Development

Neuroendocrine changes during puberty result in growth of most organ systems and alterations in body composition, blood pressure, serum lipids, and various metabolic parameters (9–14). Since adolescents enter puberty at different ages and develop at different rates, estimating the level of physical development is necessary for accurate assessment of body measurements and laboratory values. For example, serum lipids typically dip during early adolescent growth before rising again (12–14). Normative values of serum cholesterol will, therefore, vary among adolescents of the same age depending on their level of pubertal development. Likewise, other measurements, such as blood pressure, are also more dependent on physical development than on chronological age.

Psychosocial Development

Adolescence is a time during which youth develop expanded cognitive capabilities and a more well-defined self-identity. As a result of these processes adolescents begin to make an increasing number of personal decisions that are independent of direct parental influences. Adolescents also begin to assume expanded social roles within the family and the community (15–17). These changes have several implications for clinical preventive services.

First, since the ability to understand complex health concepts evolves developmentally, physicians need to ensure that their clinical interview and health guidance are geared at the appropriate conceptual level of the individual (18–21). If approached at a conceptual level that is too low, adolescents might perceive that the physician is "talking down" to them; but if the approach is too complex, the adolescent might not understand the questions or the information discussed. Second, evolving psychosocial maturity also requires that physicians judge the degree to which parents should be involved in the preventive intervention directed at the adolescent. The need for parental involvement is clearly different for 11–14-year-old adolescents than it is for adolescents between 18 and 21. Third, as adolescents develop greater psychosocial maturity, the nature of the physician-patient relationship needs to change from the authoritarian style used with children to the authoritative style used with adults. Involving adolescents more actively in formulating a management plan helps them assume greater responsibility for their health and increases their compliance.

Cultural, Ethnic, and Racial Differences

With the increasing diversity of American society, cultural, ethnic, and racial differences between physicians and their adolescent patients are more common. Distrust of the provider, stereotypical and prejudicial views of minority adolescents, inability to understand a racial minority's unique problems—these are just a few of the difficulties faced by adolescents and physicians from different backgrounds. Physicians must be aware, for example, that psychosocial development may be especially difficult for minority adolescents who, on the one hand, are faced with societal prejudice and, on the other, must incorporate their cultural heritage into a personal identity (22). Failure by physicians to recognize and understand these differences can lead to misdiagnosis, lack of cooperation, noncompliance, poor use of health services, and a general alienation of the adolescent from the health care system (23). There is growing expert opinion that physicians need to recognize individual differences and organize their practices to work effectively with culturally diverse populations (22, 24).

CONFIDENTIAL SERVICES

Justification

"Confidentiality refers to the privileged and private nature of information provided during the health care transaction" (25). Although ensuring confidentiality of the information exchanged during a preventive service visit is relatively straightforward for adults, for adolescents it is complicated by the issue of whether they can legally provide informed consent for the intervention.

"Informed consent means that the individual can understand the risks and benefits of the proposed treatment and treatment alternatives, and decide voluntarily whether to proceed with the physician's recommendations" (25, 26). Although state law does not, in general, recognize the legal rights of minors, many states allow emancipated or mature minors to provide informed consent for general health services. Emancipated minors include youths under legal age who are married, serving in the military, or living away from home and managing their own financial affairs (27, 28). Mature minors are adolescents under the age of 21 who, though living at home, demonstrate the cognitive maturity to understand the risks and benefits of a proposed medical treatment and its alternatives, and who can voluntarily decide whether to undergo treatment (29). Many states also permit minors to consent to specific medical services. These services include diagnosis of pregnancy and prenatal care, contraceptive services, diagnosis and treatment for STDs, and alcohol and drug treatment (30). Preventive interventions recommended by GAPS address many of these services. It is worth noting that there have been no known cases in which a physician has been successfully sued for providing non-negligent treatment to an adolescent over the age of 14 without parental consent (31).

Justification for this recommendation is based on two lines of evidence. The first reflects strong national consensus endorsing confidential health services for adolescents. In a recent review of health policies of national health organizations, Gans found 12 of 22 membership organizations surveyed had a policy that directly supported adolescents' need for confidential services (30). The remaining 10 organizations had no related policy; no organizations had policy counter to this concept. Major national commission reports released over the past several years also support confidential health services for adolescents. These include: *Turning Points*, produced by the Carnegie Council on Adolescent Development; *Code Blue: Uniting for Healthier Youth*, produced by the National Commission on the Role of the School and the Community in Promoting Adolescent Health (a joint effort of the National Association of State Boards of Education and the AMA); and *Adolescent Health* by the Congressional Office of Technology Assessment (32–34).

Data from various studies indicate that most practicing physicians also support confidential health services for adolescents. Lovett and Wald surveyed a random sample of 932 pediatricians and presented them with four vignettes describing case histories of adolescent females seeking confidential health services (35). The problems included a request for contraceptives, the diagnosis and treatment of gonorrhea, the disclosure of illicit drug use, and an IUD found incidentally on x-ray examination. Fifty-eight percent of physicians reported that they would provide confidential health care to adolescents in all four vignettes, while 75% would do so in one or more of the vignettes. Only 4% reported that they would not provide confidential services in any of the four situations presented. Physicians were more likely to offer confidential health services to older and more mature adolescents, and to those who wanted contraceptive services as opposed to treatment for substance abuse. Younger physicians were more likely to provide confidential services than were older physicians.

A 1987 national AMA survey of over 600 physicians (family physicians, pediatricians, and obstetricians-gynecologists) also found strong physician support for adolescent confidential health care (36). Physicians in this survey were also more likely to favor confidential health services for older rather than younger adolescents. Thirty-nine percent of physicians supported the need for confidential health services for 12–14-year-old adolescents, while 63% supported these services for 15–17-year-olds. Finally, Resnick and associates, in a survey of 500 physicians practicing in the midwest found that 75% favored confidential treatment of adolescents (37). Forty-five percent supported confidential health services unconditionally, while 30% supported confidential services with some conditions. Support for confidentiality was associated with the belief that adolescents have special needs, and with the physician's age, experience treating adolescents with sexual and interpersonal problems, and feelings of competence in managing adolescent sexual issues.

The second line of evidence for this recommendation is based on data underscoring the central role of confidentiality in the use of adolescent health services. Based on data from 170 focus groups comprising more than 800 high school students, Resnick and associates reported that confidentiality emerged as a central theme in what adolescents considered important in the delivery of health care (38). Their reasons included the need to prevent rumors and embarrassment, to avoid retribution from punitive parents, and to find a means for enhancing problem-solving abilities. Confidentiality is acknowledged to be ". . . essential to a patient's trust in a health care provider and to a patient's willingness to supply information candidly for his or her benefit" (39). This trust, in turn, facilitates the adolescent's willingness to provide accurate and frank information.

Physicians and adolescents alike believe uncertainty about confidentiality of health services leads some youths to suppress relevant information and to delay or avoid medical care (26, 38, 40, 41). Marks and associates, in a study of suburban youth, found that if parental notification were required, only 45% of adolescents reported that they would seek services for depression, 19% for birth control, 15% for treatment for a STD, and 17% for treatment of drug use (40). If assured confidentiality, however, these figures rose substantially: 57% reported that they would seek care for depression, 64% for contraceptive services, 65% for STDs, and 66% for drug use. Friedman and associates interviewed 54 adolescent substance abusers about their previous medical encounters (41). Almost all adolescents reported that they had seen a physician during the past year. Only 57%, however, recalled having been asked about substance use. Of these, almost half lied about their use of drugs, predominantly because a parent was present when the question was asked. In a recently reported study, Cheng and associates studied confidential health concerns and care-seeking behavior among 1,295 students in the 9th through 12th grades (42). Forty percent of students (55% of males and 64% of females) stated they have health concerns that they would not want their parents to know about, and 25% of students (21% of males and 29% of females) reported that they would not seek health care because of fear their parents would find out. Although over 54% had never discussed confidentiality with their physician, 64% of adolescents thought that a physician's office offered better privacy than did other clinical sites. Concern with confidentiality also may influence where adolescents go for their health services. For example, Fisher and associates found that 77% of 180 suburban adolescent patients cited confidentiality as the major reason they chose to seek medical care from a university adolescent health clinic (43). Also, in a study of 31 family planning clinics in eight cities, Chamie and associates found that 70% of white and 39% of black adolescents reported that concern about confidentiality was one of the reasons they chose to attend a community clinic rather than go to their private physician for contraceptive services (44). In summary, the results of these studies underscore two points: (1) the need for physicians to explicitly communicate to adolescent patients their office policy regarding confidentiality and (2) the opportunities physicians have to improve adolescent access to care by ensuring privacy.

Clinical Application

GAPS is designed as a health care package beyond traditional acute and chronic health care services. For preventive services to be effective, they must be delivered on an annual basis, they must be individualized, and they must be provided in a confidential manner.

Adolescents are a developmentally heterogenous group who are exposed to a variety of different risk factors. Content and delivery style appropriate for one adolescent might not be appropriate for another. Physicians will need to tailor the content of their health guidance and screening and the degree to which parents are involved by the developmental level, living situation, and individual risk factors of the adolescent. This information can be obtained during the yearly clinical interview.

A major aspect of delivering individualized preventive services is ensuring that the care provided is sensitive to and appropriate for the adolescent's cultural and ethnic background. Providing this type of service includes assessing the individual's health care needs in relation to his or her cultural group; honoring and respecting cultural beliefs, values, and family styles; and recognizing that each family represents a unique combination of economic status, religion, and ethnicity (22).

Confidentiality is critical to ensure that adolescents provide accurate information about sensitive health issues. The confidential nature of the preventive service visit should be made known to adolescents and their parents. This can be done by placing a notice on the office wall and by explaining confidentiality during the initial clinical interview. Although confidential care is sometimes perceived as a contest of rights between parents and adolescents, the need for privacy is better understood when it is seen as a normal part of development.

References

1. Gans JE, Blyth DA, Elster AB, Gaveras LL. America's Adolescents: How Healthy Are They? Chicago: American Medical Association, 1990.

2. US Department of Education. Youth Indicators 1991: Trends in the Well-Being of American Youth. Washington, DC: US Government Printing Office. PIP 91–863, 1991.

3. Bachman JG, Johnston LD, O'Malley PM. Monitoring the Future: Questionnaire Responses From the Nation's High School Seniors 1988. Ann Arbor, MI: Institute for Social Research, 1991.

4. The Alan Guttmacher Institute. Facts in Brief: Teenage Sexual and Reproductive Behavior. New York: The Alan Guttmacher Institute, 1992.

5. Zabin L, Kanter J, Zelnick M. The risk of adolescent pregnancy in the first months of intercourse. Fam Plann Perspect 1979;11:215–222.

6. Hofferth S, Hayes C, eds. Risking the Future: Adolescent Sexuality, Pregnancy, and Childbearing (Vol. 2). Washington, DC: National Academy Press, 1987.

7. Mosher W, McNally J. Contraceptive use at first marital intercourse: United States, 1965–1988. Fam Plann Perspect 1991;23:108–116.

8. Grant WW, Fearnow RG, Hebertson LM, Henderson AL. Health screening in school-age children: the physician and paramedical personnel. Am J Dis Child 1973;125:520–522.

9. Daniel W. Hematocrit: maturity relationships in adolescents. Pediatrics 1973;52:388–394.

10. Lauer R, Burns T, Clarke W. Assessing children's blood pressure. Considerations of age and body size. Pediatrics 1985;75:1081–1090.

11. Weir M, Stafford E, Gregory G. The relationship between sexual maturity rating, age, and increased blood pressure in adolescents. J Adolesc Health Care 1988;9:465–469.

12. US Department of Health and Human Services, NIH. Lipid Research Clinics Population Studies Data Book, Volume I: The Prevalence Study. Washington, DC: USDHHS, NIH Publication 80–1527, 1980.

13. Freedman D, Cresanta J. Longitudinal serum lipoprotein changes in white males during adolescence: the Bogalusa Heart Study. Metabolism 1985;34:396–403.

14. Laskarzewski P, Morrison J, et al. High and low density lipoprotein cholesterol in adolescent boys: relationships with endogenous testosterone, estradiol, and Quetelet index. Metabolism 1983;32:262–271.

15. Daniels J. Adolescent separation-individuation and family transitions. Adolescence 1990;25:105–116.

16. Newman B. The changing nature of the parent-child relationship from early to late adolescence. Adolescence 1989;24:915–924.

17. Hill J, Hombeck G, Marlow L, Green T, Lynch M. Pubertal status and parent-child relations in families of seventh-grade boys. J Early Adolesc 1985;5:31–44.

18. Bibace R, Walsh M. Development of children's concepts of illness. Pediatrics 1980;66:912–917.

19. Chassin L, Presson C, Sherman S. Applications of social development psychology to adolescent health behaviors. In: Eisenberg N, ed. Contemporary Topics in Developmental Psychology. New York: John Wiley & Sons, 1987:353–374.

20. Dielman T, Leech S, Becker M, Rosenstock I, Horvath W. Dimensions of children's health beliefs. Health Educ Q 1980; 7:219–238.

21. Mickalide A. Children's understanding of health and illness: implications for health promotion. Health Values 1986;10:5–21.

22. Voegtle K, Davis B. Meeting the Health Care Needs of Culturally Diverse Youth. Chicago: American Medical Association, 1993 (in press).

23. Nidorf J, Morgan M. Cross cultural issues in adolescent medicine. Prim Care 1987;14:69–82.

24. Bazron B, Dennis K, Isaacs M. Toward a Culturally Competent System of Care: A Monograph on Effective Services for Minority Children Who Are Severely Emotionally Disturbed. Washington, DC: Child and Adolescent Service Program (CASSP) Technical Assistance Center, Georgetown University Child Development Center, 1987.

25. AMA Council on Scientific Affairs. Confidential health services for adolescents. JAMA 1993;269:1420–1424.

26. Hofmann AD. A rational policy toward consent and confidentiality in adolescent health care. J Adolesc Health Care 1980;1:9–17.

27. English A. Ensuring access to health care for teenagers: legal and ethical issues concerning consent and confidentiality. Youth Law News 1985;4/5:22–24.

28. Morrissey JM, Hofmann AD, Thorpe JC. Consent and Confidentiality in the Health Care of Children and Adolescents: A Legal Guide. New York: The Free Press, 1986.

29. Gittler J, Quigley-Rich M, Saks MJ. Adolescent Health Care Decision-Making: The Law and Public Policy. New York: Carnegie Corporation, 1990.

30. Gans JE. Policy Compendium on Confidential Health Services for Adolescents. Chicago: American Medical Association, 1993.

31. Holder AR. Disclosure and consent problems in pediatrics. Law Med Health Care 1988;16:219–228.

32. Carnegie Council on Adolescent Development. Turning Points: Preparing American Youth for the Twenty-First Century. New York: Carnegie Foundation, 1989.

33. The National Commission on the Role of the School and the Community in Improving Adolescent Health. Code Blue: Uniting for Healthier Youth. Chicago: American Medical Association, 1989.

34. US Congress, Office of Technology Assessment. Adolescent Health-Volume I: Summary and Policy Options. OTA-H-468. Washington, DC: US Government Printing Office, April 1991.

35. Lovett J, Wald MS. Physician attitudes toward confidential care for adolescents. J Pediatr 1985;106:517–521.

36. Harvey LK, Shubat SC. Physician Opinion on Health Care Issues: 1987. Chicago: American Medical Association, 1988.

37. Resnick MD, Litman TJ, Blum RW. Physician attitudes toward confidentiality of treatment for adolescents: findings from the Upper Midwest Regional Physicians Survey. J Adolesc Health 1992;13:616–622.

38. Resnick MD, Blum RW, Hedin D. The appropriateness of health services for adolescents: youths' opinions and attitudes. J Adolesc Health Care 1980;1:137–141.

39. National Conference of Commissioners on Uniform State Laws. Uniform Health Care Information Act, Uniform Laws Annotated, Part I. St. Paul, MN: West Publishing Co, 1988:475–520.

40. Marks A, Malizio J, Hoch J, Brody R, Fisher M. Assessment of health needs and willingness to utilize health care resources of adolescents in a suburban population. J Pediatr 1983;102:456–460.

41. Friedman L, Johnson B, Brett A. Evaluation of substance-abusing adolescents by primary care physicians. J Adolesc Health Care 1990;11:227–230.

42. Cheng TL, Savageau JA, DeWitt TG. Confidentiality in health care: A survey of knowledge, perceptions, and attitudes among high school students. JAMA 1993;269:1404–1407.

43. Fisher M, Marks A, Trieller K, Brody R. Are adolescents able and willing to pay the fee for confidential health care? J Pediatr 1985;170:480–483.

44. Chamie M, Eisman S, Forrest JD, Orr MT, Torres A. Factors affecting adolescents' use of family planning clinics. Fam Plann Perspect 1982;14:126–139.

CHAPTER 2

Rationale and Recommendation: Parenting and Family Adjustment

PREVENTION STRATEGY

GAPS recommends that parents or other adult caregivers of adolescents should receive health guidance at least one time during early adolescence (i.e., age 11–14), one time during middle adolescence (i.e., age 15–17), and preferably, one time during late adolescence (i.e., age 18–21). Health guidance should focus on helping parents adjust to the changing needs of their adolescents. The broad nature of this recommendation reflects the central role that parents have in promoting adolescent development, health, and well-being. In addition to the benefits of improved family communication and relationships, health guidance for families may help reduce the risk of intentional and unintentional injuries; use of tobacco products, alcohol, and other abusable substances; and unsafe sexual practices. The concept of providing anticipatory guidance to parents of infants is accepted medical practice; GAPS extends this concept to parents of adolescents. Physician guidelines for promoting parenting and family adjustment are addressed by GAPS Recommendation 4.

DISCUSSION

The physical, emotional, and behavioral changes experienced by adolescents have an impact on, and in turn are influenced by, the broader family environment. Families are also faced with making significant adjustments throughout their child's adolescence (1–4). During puberty there is an increase in the emotional distance between adolescents and their parents; there is also an increase in adolescents' social influence within the family (3, 4). Although most families adapt to changing relationships without much difficulty, these normative changes usually lead to some degree of stress and family conflict. Parent-adolescent conflicts appear to increase during early adolescence, remain at this level during middle adolescence, and decline in frequency during late adolescence (1–4). Conflicts most frequently are over a small number of issues (e.g., chores, curfews, and other indicators of rights or responsibilities) that do not include "hot" topics such as sexual behavior, religion, drug use, or political beliefs. Although stressful, a limited amount of parent-adolescent conflicts may actually be healthy for personal development and are not associated with adverse consequences. Much less studied are the changes in family dynamics that occur as older youth either leave the home or establish an independent living arrangement within the home. These situations are also probably associated with significant adjustments in family roles and responsibilities.

Because families are the predominant socializing agent for children, they also exert the predominant influence on health behaviors. Parents influence adolescent attitudes and behaviors in at least three ways: through their modeling of health behaviors, through their health beliefs and how clearly these are expressed, and through their efforts at actively educating or training adolescents about health issues. Of these three mechanisms, role modeling appears to exert the strongest effect (5). Although youths are increasingly influenced in their attitudes and behaviors by other social influences—such as peer groups, mass media, and other adults—the effects of parents remain strong (5, 6). Lau and associates present a socialization model that ". . . predicts that parental influence on children's health beliefs and behavior generally will persist throughout life unless the child is exposed during certain critical periods to important social models whose health beliefs and behavior differ from those of the parents" (5). Critical "periods of vulnerability" include early and middle adolescence when autonomy develops, late adolescence when youth leave the home, and the time when youth establish their own home with a partner. It is at these times, Lau and associates propose, that ". . . individuals are particularly open to influence from socializing agents other than the parents."

JUSTIFICATION

What is the Association Between Parenting Behaviors, Parental Monitoring, and Adolescent Development?

Although parents may differ in their approach to rearing children, three parenting styles can be distinguished based upon ways in which parents emotionally respond to their adolescents and the manner in which they enforce discipline (7, 8). These styles are: (1) an authoritative parenting style, which is distinguished by high levels of parental warmth, support, and reasoning—and by a high level of discipline; (2) an authoritarian style, which is distinguished by high levels of discipline, but relatively low levels of warmth and reasoning; and (3) a permissive style, which is distinguished by a relatively high level of emotional responsiveness coupled with a low level of discipline. Compared to their peers, adolescents reared by authoritative parents express a greater degree of self-confidence and are more likely to engage in behaviors that are considered "normal" or "healthy," such as better school performance, greater self-reliance, less psychological stress, and less experimentation with tobacco, alcohol, or illegal substances (7–14).

Possible reasons for these findings are that adolescents raised in families with a high level of effective communication and a high level of discipline may be more aware of their parents' health beliefs, may be more willing to maintain parental standards, and may be less receptive to other social influences than are adolescents raised in families with other social dynamics. Although there is a question of how well the relation between parenting style and health-risk behavior generalizes to all adolescents, results of recent studies suggest that this association may be consistent across gender, racial and ethnic groups, and family structure (8, 9). Some experts express the opinion, however, that an authoritarian approach may be socially protective for adolescents who live in physically dangerous environments where youth are routinely exposed to drugs and violence (8, 9).

Another important dimension of parental behavior that influences adolescent development is the monitoring of social behaviors. Effective monitoring does not necessitate intrusion or require that parents always be present, but it does imply that parents have an active interest in their adolescents' social and recreational behaviors, peer group composition, and academic achievement (15). Consistent monitoring of adolescents by parents or other adults is difficult in contemporary society because of the large number of families in which both parents work outside the home, the large number of single-parent families, and the high frequency of family relocations which disrupt social networks.

Research data on the effect of parental monitoring provide a consistent finding: regardless of socioeconomic family background, a lack of parental monitoring, especially in regard to after-school care, is associated with involvement in problem behaviors and susceptibility to peer pressure (16–18). Adolescents from single-parent families are more at risk for engaging in problem behavior, possibly because there is generally less parental monitoring, less setting of limits, and less parental control in this type of family structure than in two-parent families (11, 14). Lack of appropriate monitoring may not only permit adolescents to experiment with adverse health behaviors without parental knowledge, but it also may permit adolescents to continue their association with a deviant peer group.

Additional aspects of parental monitoring include helping adolescents prevent injury and early identification of disease. Parents can ensure that the home environment is safe from firearms, that adolescents have access to a motor vehicle only when they are physically and emotionally ready, and that adolescents who participate in athletics are provided appropriate safety devices.

Despite growing evidence supporting the role of parents and the ways in which parental behavior influences adolescent development and behavior, there has been surprisingly little research or clinical attention directed at office-based anticipatory guidance for parents of otherwise healthy adolescents. Most interventions involving parents are sponsored by community organizations or target interventions for families with special health needs. For example, Small described a group of community prevention programs directed at improving parenting skills and teaching parents how to help their adolescents avoid problems with substances, alcohol, and sexual behavior (19). Although these programs demonstrate some promising results, their small and selective samples and the lack of formal evaluations make it difficult to generalize findings to other communities or settings.

DeMarsh and Kumpfer, in a review of family-oriented interventions for the prevention of substance abuse, describe a variety of programs developed to teach parents appropriate ways to manage their children and adolescents with problem behavior, to promote their child's self-esteem, and to improve family communication and problem solving (20). These programs usually targeted dysfunctional families, or parents with children and adolescents who were already involved in problem behavior. DeMarsh and Kumpfer concluded that parent training programs involving multiple group sessions may be effective in decreasing problem behavior and increasing school performance, self esteem, and communication. Other preventive interventions involving both parents and adolescents to reduce risk factors associated with cardiovascular disease have demonstrated greater success than interventions directed solely at adolescents (21–24).

What Health Guidance Do Parents Want Regarding Their Adolescents?

The second source of information justifying this recommendation comes from research suggesting that parents are deeply concerned about the current health status of adolescents and want information and guidance. Cohen and associates assessed parental reactions to the onset of adolescence in a diverse sample of 400 families (25). Parents identified four types of changes in their

young adolescents: perceived positive changes, such as being more depend-
able and more moral; perceived negative interpersonal changes, such as
being more temperamental and more bossy; perceived changes in body
awareness, such as heightened interest in clothes and appearance; and perceived negative behavioral changes, such as being more hesitant to obey
family rules and being less reliable. In response to these changes, parents
expressed a range of feelings, including feelings of confusion and being out
of control; feelings of happiness and pride; and feelings of anxiety and worry.
Younger parents (i.e., those less than age 39) in comparison to older parents
tended to have more negative perceptions of adolescent changes and to have
more negative feelings and more anxiety. Single parents perceived more positive changes among their adolescents than did parents from two-parent
households.

In another study, Fisher surveyed 438 parents, predominantly from
upper-middle-class socioeconomic backgrounds, to determine their views of
adolescent health (26). These parents expressed a high level of concern for
behavioral and psychosocial health problems of their adolescents. They also
reported a high level of interest in receiving help from their schools and their
physicians in dealing with these problems. Health issues identified as needing
the greatest attention were problems with substance use, sexuality, and mental health disorders; interest in nutrition and general medical issues rated
somewhat lower in priority. Most parents thought physicians should discuss
these health issues routinely with their adolescent patients, and that this
should occur before age 14.

Cavanaugh and associates surveyed 932 parents of adolescents seen in
pediatrician offices to assess their opinions regarding anticipatory guidance
for adolescents (27). Parents were presented a list of 30 health issues including traditional medical topics, such as acne and nutrition; behavioral topics,
such as smoking and drinking, safe sex, and discipline; and emotional topics,
such as depression, family relationships, and eating disorders. As in the study
by Fisher, parents expressed a high level of interest in having these health
issues discussed with their adolescents. Thus, 24 of the 30 health issues were
judged by at least 75% of parents as important enough to include in routine
health guidance. These rates differed by both age and gender of the adolescent. The results of other studies also support the conclusion that parents
are concerned about the psychosocial and behavioral issues of their children
and adolescents, and that they look to physicians for guidance (28, 29).
Finally, the results from a series of studies by Webster and associates suggest
there is strong support from both parents and physicians regarding the need
and the desire to have health guidance on handgun safety provided during

clinical visits (30, 31). Approximately 90% of parents reported they would be willing to disclose to physicians that they owned a handgun, and 75% stated they would comply with their physician's recommendation to keep guns unloaded and locked (31).

CLINICAL INTERVENTION

Health guidance for parents provided in a clinical setting is viewed by expert opinion as an important component of a strategy to help adolescents adopt healthy lifestyles and reduce their risk of premature morbidity and mortality. Although time restraints of clinical practice prohibit a lengthy intervention, parents can be provided information, guidance, and encouragement that may help them respond to the health needs of their adolescents. For example, investigators have found that parents who recalled seeing or hearing public service announcements (PSA) on AIDS, or reading an AIDS brochure, were more likely to discuss AIDS with their children than were other parents (69% versus 53% for reading the PSA; 76% versus 57% for reading a brochure; and 66% versus 58% for hearing a PSA) (32).

The results of this study imply that increased awareness of health problems may promote parent-adolescent discussions about health-risk behaviors. These discussions may provide adolescents a clearer expression of parental values and expectations which, in turn, provide guidance to adolescents when they need to make decisions regarding involvement in health-risk behaviors. Other ways to provide parents' with information and guidance without using excessive provider time include sponsoring group educational sessions, having audiovisual and printed material available in the office, and having parents counseled by other office personnel. Completing a previsit checklist asking about behavioral concerns is another method that conserves office time and promotes improved communication between parents and physicians (33).

REFERENCES

1. Hill JP, Holmbeck GN, Marlow L, Green TM, Lynch ME. Pubertal status and parent-child relations in families of seventh-grade boys. J Early Adolesc 1985;5:31–44.
2. Paikoff RL, Brooks-Gunn J. Do parent-child relationships change during puberty? Psychol Bull 1991;110:47–66.
3. Newman B. The changing nature of the parent-child relationship from early to late adolescence. Adolescence 1989;96:915–924.

4. Montemayor R. Parents and adolescents in conflict: all families some of the time and some families most of the time. J Early Adolesc 1983;3:83–103.

5. Lau RR, Quadrel MJ, Hartman KA. Development and change of young adults' preventive health beliefs and behavior: influence of parents and peers. J Health Soc Behav 1990;31:240–259.

6. Hansell S, Mechanic D. Parent and peer effects on adolescent health behavior. In: Hurrelmann K, Losel F, eds. Health Hazards in Adolescence. New York: Walter de Gruyter, 1990:43–65.

7. Baumrind D. A developmental perspective on adolescent risk-taking in contemporary America. In: Irwin CE, ed. New Directions for Child Development: Adolescent Social Behavior and Health. San Francisco: Jossey-Bass, 1987:92–126.

8. Steinberg L, Mounts NS, Lamborn SD, Dornbusch SM. Authoritative parenting and adolescent adjustment across varied ecological niches. J Res Adolesc 1991;1:19–36.

9. Dornbusch SM, Ritter PL, Leiderman PH, Roberts DF, Fraleigh MJ. The relation of parenting style to adolescent school performance. Child Dev 1987;58:1244–1257.

10. Barnes GM. Adolescent alcohol abuse and other problem behaviors: their relationships and common parental influences. J Youth Adolesc 1984;13:329–348.

11. Turner RA, Irwin CE, Millstein SG. Family structure, family processes, and experimenting with substances during adolescence. J Res Adolesc 1991;1:93–106.

12. Baumrind D. Parenting styles and adolescent development. In: Lerner RM, Peterson AC, Brooks-Gunn J, eds. Encyclopedia of Adolescence. New York: Garland, 1991:746–758.

13. Dishion TJ, Patterson GR, Reid JR. Parent and peer factors associated with drug sampling in early adolescence: implication for treatment. In: Adolescent Drug Abuse: Analyses of Treatment Research. NIDA Research Monograph Series 77, 1988. DHHS Publication (ADM) 69–93.

14. Dishion TJ, Loeber R. Adolescent marijuana and alcohol use: the role of parents and peers revisited. Am J Drug Alcohol Abuse 1985;11:11–25.

15. Small SA, Eastman G. Rearing adolescents in contemporary society: a conceptual framework for understanding the responsibilities and needs of parents. Fam Relations 1991;40:455–462.

16. Steinberg L. Latchkey children and susceptibility to peer pressure: an ecological analysis. Dev Psychol 1986;22:433–439.

17. Richardson JL, Dwyer K, McGuigan K, et al. Substance use among eighth-grade students who take care of themselves after school. Pediatrics 1989;84:556–566.

18. Dwyer KM, Richardson JL, Danley KL, et al. Characteristics of eighth-grade students who initiate self-care in elementary and junior high school. Pediatrics 1990;86:448–454.

19. Small S. Preventive programs that support families with adolescents. Working paper prepared for the Carnegie Council on Adolescent Development. Washington, DC: Carnegie Corporation, 1990.

20. DeMarsh J, Kumpfer KL. Family-oriented interventions for the prevention of chemical dependency in children and adolescents. Child Contem Soc 1985;18:117–151.

21. Perry CL, Luepker RV, Murray DM, et al. Parent involvement with children's health promotion: the Minnesota home team. Am J Public Health 1988;78:1156–1160.

22. Perry CL, Brockett SJ, Pirie P. Influencing parental health behavior: implications of community assessments. Health Educ Q 1987;18:68–77.

23. Coates T, Killen J, Slinkard L. Parent participation in a treatment program for overweight adolescents. Int J Eat Disorders 1982;1:37–47.

24. BrownellK, Kelman J, Stunkard A. Treatment of obese children with and without their mothers: changes in weight and blood pressure. Pediatrics 1983;71:515–523.

25. Cohen M, Adler N, Beck A, Irwin CE. Parental reactions to the onset of adolescence. J Adolesc Health Care 1986;7:101–106.

26. Fisher M: Parents' views of adolescent health issues. Pediatrics 1992;90:335–341.

27. Cavanaugh RM, Hasting-Tolsma M, Keenan D, Henneberger PK. Anticipatory guidance for the adolescent: parental concerns. Clin Pediatr, 1993 (in press).

28. Stickler GB, Salter M, Broughton DD, Alario A. Parents' worries about children compared to actual risks. Clin Pediatr 1991;30:522–528.

29. Hickson GB, Altemeier WA, O'Connor S. Concerns of mothers seeking care in private pediatric offices: opportunities for expanding services. Pediatrics 1983;72:619–624.

30. Webster DW, Wilson MEH, Duggan AK, Pakula LC. Firearm injury prevention counseling: a study of pediatricians' beliefs and practices. Pediatrics 1992;89:902–907.

31. Webster DW, Wilson MEH, Duggan AK, Pakula LC. Parents' beliefs about preventing gun injuries to children. Pediatrics 1992;89:908–914.

32. Centers for Disease Control. Characteristics of parents who discuss AIDS with their children—United States, 1989. MMWR 1991;40:789–791.

33. Triggs EG, Perrin EC: Listening carefully. Improving communication about behavior and development. Clin Pediatr 1989;28:185–192.

CHAPTER 3

Rationale and Recommendation: Promoting Psychosocial Adjustment

PREVENTION STRATEGY

GAPS recommends a primary prevention strategy to help promote adolescent psychosocial and psychosexual adjustment. This strategy includes providing all adolescents with health guidance on an annual basis to help them learn how to cope with the physical, emotional, and behavioral challenges of adolescence. Important to this process is the need for adolescents to be actively involved in decisions regarding their health care. The physician guidelines for providing health guidance to adolescents are addressed in GAPS Recommendation 5.

DISCUSSION

Adolescence is a time of both emotional vulnerability and educational opportunity. It is an inherently stressful time of life during which the interaction of rapid physical, emotional, cognitive, and social changes leads to a redefining of who one is and what one wants to be in life. During this process, most adolescents develop an increasing degree of personal autonomy, a greater reliance on peer group networks for social support, a vocational goal, a more well-defined self-identify, and increasing empathy and understanding of their role in the larger world around them (1, 2). As part of their normal development, adolescents will often experiment with some type of health-risk behavior. From a prevention perspective, it is important to recognize that most adolescents who intermittently engage in health-risk behaviors are usually well-adjusted emotionally.

In association with individual physical and psychosocial changes, adolescence also changes family dynamics and increases family conflict (3–7). Furthermore, exposure to more complex peer group interactions as well as greater academic demands are also part of normal adolescent development. The types of daily stresses experienced by adolescents have a developmental

21

trajectory. Family stressors are prominent among adolescents 12–14 years old, peer relationships are the predominant stressors for adolescents 15–17 years old, and academic concerns are the major cause of stress for adolescents 18–20 years old (5).

In addition to daily stresses or "hassles" related to family and peer relationships and school performance, adolescents experience a series of expected or normative life events that also cause emotional stress. One such event is puberty. Although individual pubertal events, such as menarche or first ejaculation may cause relatively little stress (8–12), the age at which a person enters puberty in relation to his or her peer group does appear to affect emotional adjustment. Adolescents who develop "on time" with their peer group have a somewhat easier time emotionally than do adolescents who develop either early or late (13–15). Another major normative life event is making the transition to a higher level of school, such as moving from elementary to junior high (or middle) school (16, 17). School transitions expose adolescents to more diverse peer group influences in a social environment that is larger, less individualized, and less capable of providing adult supervision and social support. Some adolescents may have difficulty coping with this larger, more impersonal social environment, especially if they are troubled by other events in their life. Promising results have been found from studies of programs offered through schools to help young adolescents with transition to middle school (5). Still other normative life events that necessitate social adaptation include the onset of dating and family relocation.

Adolescents may also experience unexpected, or non-normative stressful life events, of which divorce is one of the most common. Over one million children are involved in divorces each year. In addition to the socioeconomic effects on the custodial family, divorce during childhood can lead to emotional problems during adolescence, especially when divorce is followed by remarriage (18–20). Hetherington and associates have found that, at least with younger children, divorce has a more adverse effect on boys, while remarriage of a custodial mother is more problematic for girls (19). Peterson and Zill, in an analysis of a national sample of 1,400 children 12 to 16 years of age, found that marital disruption was associated with a range of negative outcomes for both boys and girls (20). In support of the previous work of Hetherington, Peterson and Zill found that remarriage had a differential effect, depending on the gender of the teenager and the custodial parent (19).

Interventions provided in school and community programs have been used to help adolescents and their families cope with parental divorce and remarriage. These programs offer adolescents protective skills to deal with the stresses that result from changing marital status. In a review of these programs, Compas found that they were relatively effective in assisting children, adolescents, and their families adjust to changing family situations (5).

Adolescents usually cope with normative life events without much difficulty. Offer has demonstrated, with a range of different adolescent populations, that most youths progress through adolescence with only a minimal amount of emotional turbulence, and that this period of life is not necessarily associated with "storm and stress," as once believed (21). Some adolescents, however, do have difficulty coping and exhibit emotional distress, especially when multiple normative events occur simultaneously and are combined with non-normative life events (16, 17, 22). Gender differences in how well adolescents adjust to challenges do occur. For example, girls appear to have a somewhat more difficult time coping with adolescence than do boys, especially girls who enter puberty earlier than their age peers (5, 6, 23).

Although cognitive, emotional, and behavioral changes may present developmental challenges for adolescents, they also present opportunities for health guidance. Because of an increase in reasoning ability, emotional autonomy, and concern with body image, adolescents are capable of and interested in assuming greater control of their lives. Normative and non-normative life events, pregnancy scares resulting from missed menstrual periods, athletic participation, and other events are opportune times for providing preventive interventions. Because most adolescents have an identified source of medical care, and 70–90% have seen a medical provider during the previous year, medical settings are good opportunities for providing adolescents with routine health guidance (24–27).

Unfortunately, adolescents do not always receive the health guidance they want. For example, in a study of 362 college students, Joffe and associates found that few adolescents surveyed had received prior health counseling from their personal physician (28). Approximately 20% of men and 19–30% of women had received counseling on the use of cigarettes, alcohol, or drugs; approximately 10% of men and women had been counseled on use of seat belts; and approximately 20% of men and women had received counseling on STDs.

JUSTIFICATION

To What Extent Do Adolescents Want to Receive Health Guidance from Their Physicians?

Adolescence can be a time of anxiety during which youths experience physical changes, experiment with sexuality, and are exposed to the availability of tobacco, alcohol, and other drugs. They are forced to make decisions that may have immediate and long-term effects on their health and well-being. Justification for this recommendation comes predominantly from the results of studies suggesting that adolescents are concerned about the physical and psychosocial challenges they face. Adolescents want their physicians to provide information and guidance to help them make informed decisions.

Parcel and associates surveyed 3,255 high school students and found that most believed young people lacked adequate information about birth control, sex, drugs, and general health information, in addition to information about where to get health services (27). These opinions were similar among black, white, and Mexican-American students. In addition, while only 8% of adolescents indicated they did not know where to go if they had a health problem, 36% either found it difficult to get help or had no one available to answer health questions. Students expressed concern about a range of biopsychosocial problems and indicated strong interest in getting help for these concerns. Results from recent studies corroborate these earlier findings.

Sobal and associates, in a study of 831 students selected randomly from two urban high schools, found that 61% of adolescents think about their health frequently (25). Females were more likely than males and black students were more likely than white students to have a high level of concern. Only 8% reported a low level of concern. There was no difference in level of concern by grade level. In a study of 600 middle school students, Levenson and associates also found a high level of health concerns (29). Almost 30% of students in this study reported that they "worry about health a lot," while 40% "worry a lot" when they are sick.

In another study, Malus and associates studied 1,564 students between 13 and 18 years of age to determine what issues teenagers want to discuss with their physician and to what extent these discussions occurred (30). The topics students wanted to discuss most included exercise, nutrition, obesity, growth, STDs, contraception, alcohol, and drugs. There was a large discrepancy, however, between topics adolescents wanted to discuss and topics actually covered. Thus, although 80–90% of adolescents wanted information on nutrition, exercise, and growth, only 50% reported they had actually received counseling on these topics. Even greater discrepancies were found for the more emotionally sensitive issues of STDs, contraception, drugs, and alcohol.

Finally, results of a national survey by Louis Harris and Associates of 2,288 students in grades 7–12 indicate that adolescents have attitudes conducive to assuming more control over their health (24). Over 60% of adolescents believed they have control over their own health, and 73% had at some time in the past made changes to improve their health. The changes most often mentioned were related to increasing exercising and improving diet.

CLINICAL INTERVENTION

Adolescence is a period of emotional vulnerability that also presents an opportunity for helping youths take an active role in improving their health. Puberty creates heightened interest in one's body, making educational and prevention efforts timely. As role models and sources of credible information, support, and encouragement, physicians and other health professionals can help adolescents cope with challenges they will face.

Providing health guidance to help adolescents adjust to the normal physical and emotional changes they experience is a central goal of GAPS. Because of concerns for their body and their evolving emotional autonomy, adolescents are receptive to learning about health. Concerns adolescents have about puberty, peer and family pressures, somatic complaints, and other normative issues should be used to direct the counseling. One aim of health guidance should be to help adolescents gradually assume responsibility for making health related decisions. This could include instructing adolescents about the availability and appropriate use of medical services. Health guidance will be more effective if adolescents are instructed in an authoritative manner in which the physician-patient relationship is viewed as a partnership.

REFERENCES

1. Petersen AC. Adolescent development. Annu Rev Psychol 1988;39:583–607.
2. Crockett LJ, Petersen AC. Adolescent development: health risks and opportunities for health promotion. In: Millstein SG, Petersen AC, Nightingale EO, eds. Promoting the Health of Adolescents: New Directions for the Twenty-First Century. New York: Oxford University Press, 1993.
3. Hill JP, Holmbeck GN, Marlow L, Green TM, Lynch ME. Pubertal status and parent-child relations in families of seventh-grade boys. J Early Adolesc 1985;5:31–44.
4. Paikoff RL, Brooks-Gunn J. Do parent-child relationships change during puberty? Psychol Bull 1991;110:47–66.
5. Compas BE, Phares V, Ledoux N. Stress and coping preventive interventions for children and adolescents. In: Bond LA, Compas BE, eds. Primary Prevention and Promotion in the Schools. Newbury Park, CA: Sage Publications, 1989:319–340.

6. Petersen AC, Sarigiani PA, Kennedy RE. Adolescent depression: why more girls? J Youth Adolesc 1991;20:247–271.

7. Newman B. The changing nature of the parent-child relationship from early to late adolescence. Adolescence 1989;96:915–924.

8. Gaddis A, Brooks-Gunn J. The male experience of pubertal change. J Youth Adolesc 1985;14:61–69.

9. Rierdan J, Koff E. Premenarcheal predictors of experience of menarche: a prospective study. J Adolesc Health Care 1990;11:404–407.

10. Koff E, Rierdan J, Sheingold K. Memories of menarche: age, preparation, and prior knowledge as determinants of initial menstrual experience. J Youth Adolesc 1982;11:1–9.

11. Greif EB, Ulman KJ. The psychological impact of menarche on early adolescent females: a review of the literature. Child Dev 1982;53:1413–1430.

12. Ruble DN, Brooks-Gunn J. The experience of menarche. Child Dev 1982;53:1557–1566.

13. Magnusson D, Stattin H, Allen VL. Differential maturation among girls and its relation to social adjustment: a longitudinal perspective. In: Baltes PB, Featherman DL, Lerner RM, eds. Life-Span Development and Behavior. Hillsdale, NJ: Lawrence Erlbaum, 1986:135–172.

14. Duke PM, Carlsmith JM, Jennings D, et al. Educational correlates of early and late sexual maturation in adolescence. J Pediatr 1982;100:633–637.

15. Nottelmann ED, Susman EJ, Inoff-Germain G, Cutler GB, Loriaux DL, Chrousos GP. Developmental processes in early adolescence: relationships between adolescent adjustment problems and chronological age, pubertal stage, and puberty-related serum hormone levels. J Pediatr 1987;110:473–480.

16. Simmons RG, Burgeson R, Carlton-Ford S, Blyth DA. The impact of cumulative change in early adolescence. Child Dev 1987;58:1220–1234.

17. Blyth DA, Simmons RG, Carlton-Ford S. The adjustment of early adolescents to school transitions. J Early Adolesc 1983;3:105–120.

18. Amato PR, Keith B. Parental divorce and the well-being of children: a meta-analysis. Psychol Bull 1991;110:26–46.

19. Hetherington EM, Cox M, Cox R. Long-term effects of divorce and remarriage on the adjustment of children. J Am Acad Child Psychiatry 1985;24:518–530.

20. Peterson JL, Zill N. Marital disruption, parent-child relationships, and behavior problems in children. J Marr Fam 1986;48:295–307.

21. Offer D. The Psychological World of the Teenager. New York: Basic Books, 1969.

22. Compas BE. Stress and life events during childhood and adolescence. Clin Psychol Rev 1987;7:275–302

23. Rice KG, Herman MA, Petersen AC. Coping with challenge in adolescence: a conceptual model and psycho-educational intervention. J Adolesc 1993 (in press).

24. Louis Harris and Associates. Health: You've Got to be Taught. An Evaluation of Comprehensive Health Education in American Public Schools. New York: Louis Harris and Associates, 1988.

25. Sobal J, Klein H, Graham D, Black J. Health concerns of high school students and teachers' beliefs about student health concerns. Pediatrics 1988;81:218–223.

26. Marks A, Malizio J, Hoch J, Brody R, Fisher M. Assessment of health needs and willingness to utilize health care resources of adolescents in a suburban population. J Pediatr 1983;102:456–460.

27. Parcel GS, Nader PR, Meyer MP. Adolescent health concerns, problems, and patterns of utilization in a triethnic urban population. Pediatrics 1977;60:157–164.

28. Joffe A, Radius S, Gall M. Health counseling for adolescents: what they want, what they get, and who gives it. Pediatrics 1988;82:481–485.

29. Levenson PH, Morrow JR, Pfefferbaum BJ. Attitudes toward health and illness. J Adolesc Health Care 1984;5:245–260.

30. Malus M, LaChance PA, Lamy L, Macaulay A, Vanasse M. Priorities in adolescent health care: the teenager's viewpoint. J Fam Pract 1987;25:159–162.

CHAPTER 4

Rationale and Recommendations: Intentional and Unintentional Injuries

PREVENTION STRATEGY

GAPS recommends a primary preventive strategy to reduce the risk of intentional and unintentional injuries. Annual health guidance should be directed at helping adolescents: abstain from use of alcohol and other drugs when impaired judgment can lead to injury (i.e., while driving a motor vehicle or swimming); use safety devices—including seat belts, motorcycle and bicycle helmets, and appropriate athletic protective gear; identify nonviolent ways to resolve interpersonal conflicts; avoid use of handguns and other weapons; achieve physical conditioning before engaging in vigorous exercise and undergo proper rehabilitation before resuming athletic participation. Physician guidelines for injury prevention are addressed in GAPS Recommendation 6.

DISCUSSION

Injuries can be classified as either intentional or unintentional. The former group includes suicide, homicide, and other forms of interpersonal violence; the latter group includes motor vehicle crashes, drownings, and athletic injuries. Injuries are the predominant cause of mortality and morbidity among today's youth.

Between the early 1930s and the mid-1980s, the overall mortality rate declined 67% for adolescents 10–19 years old (1, 2). This general figure, however, conceals areas of major concern. For example, although the death rate from natural causes has declined, the mortality rate from injuries has remained stable. Over 75% of deaths in 1933 were from natural causes and nearly 25% were from injuries. These figures are now almost reversed, with almost 70% of deaths due to injuries. Another trend that is not obvious

Table 4.1. Leading Causes of Injury Related Adolescent Deaths by Age, Gender and Race: Number of Deaths per 100,000 Adolescents, 1986

Group	Causes of Death			
	Motor Vehicle Crashes	Homicide	Suicide	Drowning
Ages 10 to 14				
White				
Male	4.9	1.2	2.4	2.1
Female	3.4	1.1	0.7	0.5
Black				
Male	2.9	4.6	1.5	8.3
Female	1.8	2.0	0.4	1.7
Ages 15 to 19				
White				
Male	46.5	8.5	18.2	5.6
Female	22.0	3.3	4.0	0.5
Black				
Male	18.7	50.7	7.1	11.0
Female	6.4	12.1	2.1	0.9

Source: Centers for Disease Control. Childhood injuries in the United States. Am J Dis Child, 1990; 144: 727-646.

from the overall figures is that until the early 1980s, the decline in adolescent mortality was relatively equal for all adolescents. Since then, however, the death rate among black adolescent males has risen substantially, while rates for white males and for females have remained somewhat stable (1).

Causes of injury deaths among adolescents vary substantially by age, gender, and race. The leading causes of injury-related adolescent deaths for 1986 are shown in Table 4.1 (3).

Two major conclusions can be drawn from these data. First, death rates are greater for males and for older adolescents than for females and younger adolescents. Second, among males, white youths are at greater risk of death from a motor vehicle crash and from suicide, while black youths are at greater risk of death from homicide and drowning. The table does not show that 70% of deaths from injuries and 50% of all adolescent deaths are from unintentional causes (4). Although alarming, these figures fail to account for a much larger group of adolescents who suffer severe trauma or permanent disability from injuries.

Kraus and associates reviewed data from four major studies and found that adolescents 15–19 years old suffer more traumatic brain injuries than other age groups (5). Between 300 and 600 adolescents per 100,000 suffer brain injuries each year, with rates substantially greater for males than for females. Data from one of the studies, a review of injuries from San Diego County, indicated that among adolescents 15–19, 75% of brain injuries were classified as mild, 16% were classified as severe to moderate, and 8% resulted in immediate death (5). The greatest single cause of brain injury among adolescents was motor vehicle crashes (55%), followed by assault (17%), sports or recreation (10%), and falls (9%).

Additional indication of morbidity from injury is provided by results of several studies suggesting that 1–2.5% of adolescents each year suffer an unintentional injury severe enough to require an emergency room visit; an additional 1.7–2% have an injury that is treated in a medical clinic (6, 7). However, because injury surveillance studies include only unintentional injuries, the total magnitude of the morbidity resulting from all injuries is understated.

Direct costs for the immediate and the long-term treatment of injuries contributes significantly to health care expenditures. Next to young adults 25–44 years old, adolescents incur the greatest lifetime costs from injury of any age group (8). The Centers for Disease Control and Prevention (CDC) estimated that expenses for medical treatment and rehabilitation associated with adolescent injury totalled $8.9 billion in 1985. CDC also estimated the loss of future earnings from disability as $15.7 billion and the loss from death as $14.5 billion. Adolescent injuries have a greater impact—in human suffering and in financial cost to society—than any other health condition targeted by GAPS recommendations.

JUSTIFICATION

GAPS adopts the primary prevention strategy of providing counseling to all adolescents about reducing their risk of injury. Justification for this set of recommendations comes from the large burden of suffering adolescents experience as a result of injuries and from the opportunity to use the preventive service visit to counsel adolescents about factors placing them at risk for injury.

What are the Risk Factors for Injury Among Adolescents and What Can Physicians Do to Reduce These Risks?

There are four major risk factors associated with injuries to adolescents: use of alcohol and other drugs while engaged in activities—such as driving or swimming—where impaired judgment can have serious outcomes; failure to use safety devices, such as seat belts and bicycle or motorcycle helmets; access to firearms; and participation in sports. Each of these risks represents an area for health guidance.

Alcohol and drug-related injury and death are especially prominent aspects of adolescent health, as reflected in the following statistics (2–4, 9, 10). Approximately 20% of all deaths among adolescents 15–20 years old are from alcohol-related car crashes; adolescents younger than 21 are twice as likely as any other age group to be in an alcohol-related car crash; approximately half of adolescent deaths from motor vehicle crashes are alcohol related; 29.5% of adolescent driver mortalities and 47% of all mortalities involving adolescents as drivers result from alcohol-related motor vehicle crashes; and almost 24% of fatal pedestrian or bicycle accidents among adolescents are alcohol related. Kraus and associates in their study of almost 500 adolescents with brain injury found that 51% had a measurable blood alcohol level and 40% had a level over the legal limit for driving at the time of the injury (5).

Many adolescents, unfortunately, continue to risk death and serious injury by engaging in potentially dangerous activities after drinking or using drugs. For example, the results of various studies indicate that approximately 35% of adolescent males have recently ridden with a driver who used alcohol or drugs, 35% have consumed two or more drinks prior to driving, and 15% have used alcohol or drugs while swimming or boating (11, 12). Figures for females were 40%, 22%, and 11%, respectively. Williams and associates, in a multiple-state study of over 52,000 adolescents, reported that 20% of licensed drivers who drank once during the previous month also drove on that occasion (13). This figure increased with the number of times adolescents drank; 44% of those who drank two to four times during the past month and 82% of those who drank 10 or more times reported driving after drinking. A survey conducted by the CDC found that among a somewhat older population—youths 18 to 24—15% of males and 10% of females reported driving after drinking (10).

Health providers can promote injury prevention by counseling parents to closely supervise adolescents' use of an automobile and to restrict use at high-risk times, such as late at night (14, 15). In a study of four states with curfew laws, researchers found that increased supervision lowers the number of motor vehicle crashes involving adolescents by 25–69% (15). Providers should be cautious about recommending driver education and early licensure. Robertson and Zador studied the relationship between driver education and adolescent motor vehicle fatalities in 27 states over five calendar years. They found higher death rates in states with greater proportions of 16–17-year-olds receiving high school driver education (16). Driver education courses allowed 80% of adolescents to drive before the age the of 18, the age when they otherwise would have received their licenses.

A second major risk factor for adolescent injury is failure to use safety devices, such as seat belts and helmets. The results of two large surveys of secondary school students provide similar figures for the use of safety belts and helmets (11, 17). Data from these studies suggest that fewer that 50% of adolescents wear a seat belt consistently, fewer than 60% wear a motorcycle helmet consistently, and fewer than 2% wear a bicycle helmet consistently. Although rates for seat belt use are greater for females and for older adolescents, use of helmets does not vary by age or gender. In a 1989 observational study conducted in 19 cities, seat belt use among adolescents was found to be 29%—the lowest use of any age group (18). Researchers have estimated that among adolescents 10–14 years old, 20–30% of deaths from motor vehicle crashes could have been avoided with use of seat belts; 25–30% of deaths could have been avoided with use of air bags; and over 50% of deaths could have been avoided by using helmets while riding a bicycle or motorcycle (19, 20).

The few clinical trials using office counseling to promote use of safety devices have yielded conflicting results. For example, Cushman and associates studied a preventive intervention in which physicians provided families of preadolescents with counseling and a pamphlet on using bicycle helmets (21). A telephone interview two to three weeks after intervention revealed no difference between the study group and a control group regarding their purchase of a helmet. More encouraging results were found by Logsdon and associates in their study of the effectiveness of office counseling by primary care physicians in changing health-risk behaviors. Approximately 15% of patients in the study were adolescents and young adults between 18 and 24 (22, 23). One year after the intervention, significantly more subjects in the study group than in the control group reported using seat belts on a regular basis.

The third major risk factor for injury is access to firearms. This issue has generated considerable attention because of the recent dramatic increase in adolescent deaths from firearms. Firearms are responsible for 20% of all deaths among adolescents 15–19 years old (24). During the past two decades, the death rate from firearms among adolescents 15–19 has risen 75%, from 10.1 deaths per 100,000 in 1968 to 17.7 deaths per 100,000 in 1988 (24). Males, especially black males, are at a substantially greater risk to die from firearms than are other groups of adolescents. Forty-eight percent of deaths among black adolescent males result from firearms, compared with 18% of such deaths among white adolescent males (24). Of firearm deaths among adolescents 15–19, 89% are intentional (50% from homicide and 39% from suicide). Only 8% of firearm deaths among older adolescents are unintentional. From another perspective, firearms are involved in more than 70% of adolescent male homicides (over 80% of homicide deaths among black adolescent males) and over 60% of adolescent suicides (25).

The majority of firearm deaths result from handguns. Of firearm-related deaths among adolescents, 73% of homicides and 70% of suicides involved handguns (26, 27). Because of these findings, special focus has been directed at identifying strategies for reducing adolescents' access to handguns. As reported by Christoffel, there are 60 million handguns owned privately in the United States; 25 million households have a handgun and 9 million adolescents have access to handguns (28). The results of several large studies demonstrate the easy access adolescents have to handguns and their high rate of personal ownership of handguns. Indeed, 30–40% of adolescents report that handguns are easily accessible to them (11, 29). Males, older adolescents, adolescents from racial minorities, and adolescents from lower socioeconomic status (SES) family backgrounds are more likely to have easy access to handguns than are other adolescents. Data also suggest that 6% to 9% of adolescents actually own a handgun (29–31). Ownership is more prevalent among males and adolescents from racial minorities and from lower SES family backgrounds. The median age for acquiring a handgun is during early adolescence—between the ages of 12 and 15 (29, 30). In one study, Callahan and Rivara could not distinguish adolescents who owned guns from those who did not by their participation in school sports, church membership, or employment (29). Although ownership was associated with gang membership and other conduct problems, 63% of adolescents who owned guns did not belong to a gang. Callahan and Rivara concluded that handgun ownership was not restricted to any one social class, racial group, or subpopulation of adolescents with deviant behavior.

Results of recent studies also indicate that access to handguns in the home, even when they are supposedly secured, is associated with risk for suicide (32). In another set of studies mortality data were collected from two demographically similar cities, one with a hand gun regulation and one without. For 15–19-year-olds, these data indicate that the risk of homicide from firearms is 4.8 times greater, and the risk of suicide is 1.38 times greater, in the city without a hand gun regulation (33, 34).

Providers should counsel parents on the control of firearms. Webster and associates found that 74% of pediatricians surveyed believed they have a responsibility to counsel families about firearms. Over 95% of pediatricians supported counseling families with children to keep firearms unloaded and locked, while 75% supported counseling these families to remove firearms from the home (35). Over 65% of pediatricians surveyed believed that parents are likely to heed a physician's advice about storing firearms safely and 30% believed that parents would follow their advice about not having guns in the home. In a companion study, these same investigators found that 90% of parents would be willing to tell their doctor about family ownership of a handgun, and 75% stated they would follow their physician's advice to keep guns unloaded and locked (36). Less than 20%, however, reported that they would comply with the advice to remove guns from the home. Among non-owners, 68% reported they would be less likely to purchase a handgun if counseled by their physician. These data indicate physicians perceive they have a responsibility to counsel about handguns and that they have a reasonably accurate perception of the response they would get from parents about suggesting handgun safety.

The fourth risk factor for injury is athletic participation. Sports and recreational activities are the leading cause of nonfatal injuries among adolescents (3, 19). An estimated 5–7 million adolescents participate annually in school sports, and an additional 20 million engage in recreational sports outside of school (37). Between 20% and 40% of athletes have serious enough injuries to cause them to miss a game or practice (38, 39), with the rate of injuries for males almost double that of females. The sports most associated with injuries are football and wrestling for males and gymnastics for females. The majority of some injuries, such as trauma to the knee and leg, are actually reinjuries (39). Because of this, the history of an injury and the degree of rehabilitation appear to be the best predicator of future orthopedic problems (40). Studies have compared the most commonly used methods of performing preparticipation examinations on a large number of athletes. The "station" examination approach, where different providers are each responsible for a specific part of the evaluation of an athlete, appears more effective at identifying adolescents with medical and orthopedic problems than does the mass examination approach, where one provider is responsible for doing a complete evaluation (41).

Clinical Application

Although the causes of serious injuries among adolescents are varied, physicians can focus health guidance on selected issues. Special attention should be given to providing health guidance to adolescents who drink or use drugs, who have access to or own handguns, who drive a motor vehicle, or who participate in organized athletics. There is some indication that older adolescents and young adults engage in multiple health-risk behaviors, such as drinking and driving, not wearing seat belts, and smoking (42, 43). Counseling should be directed at helping adolescents understand the relation among health-risk behaviors and motivating them to reduce their risk of injury.

Preventing injuries from sports and recreation can be promoted by ensuring that adolescents know the value of safety devices (e.g., helmets, mouth guards, etc.) and that they are motivated to use these devices regularly. Prior to participation in a sport, physicians should ensure that proper rehabilitation of an injury has occurred. When not performed as part of a preventive service visit, preparticipation athletic examinations on large groups of adolescents are best done using the "station" method (41). The opportunity should be used to screen and counsel adolescents regarding tobacco, alcohol, and other drugs, including anabolic steroids.

References

1. Fingerhut L, Kleinman J. Trends and current status in childhood mortality. Vital Health Stat 3. Washington, DC: US Department of Health and Human Services, 1989:1–44.

2. Gans JE, Blyth DA, Elster AB, Gaveras LL. American's Adolescents: How Healthy Are They? Chicago: American Medical Association, 1990.

3. Centers for Disease Control. Childhood injuries in the United States. Am J Dis Child 1990;144:646–727.

4. US Congress, Office of Technology Assessment. Adolescent Health-Volume II: Background and the Effectiveness of Selected Prevention and Treatment Services. OTA-H-466. Washington, DC: US Government Printing Office, 1991.

5. Kraus J, Rock A, Hemyari P. Brain injuries among infants, children, adolescents and young adults. Am J Dis Child 1990;144:684–691.

6. Rivara FP, Calonge N, Thompson RS. Population-based study of unintentional injury incidence and impact during childhood. Am J Public Health 1989;79:990–994.

7. Gallagher S, Finison K, Guyer B, Goodenough S. The incidence of injuries among 87,000 Massachusetts children and adolescents: results of the 1980–1981 statewide childhood injury prevention program surveillance system. Am J Public Health 1984;74:1340–1347.

8. Centers for Disease Control. Cost of injury—United States: a report to Congress, 1989. JAMA 1989;262:2803–2804.

9. National Highway Traffic Safety Administration. Fatal Accident Reporting System 1988: A Review of Information on Fatal Traffic Crashes in the United States in 1988. Washington, DC: US Department of Transportation, 1989.

10. Centers for Disease Control. Factors potentially associated with reductions in alcohol-related traffic fatalities—United States, 1990 and 1991. MMWR 1992;41:893–899.

11. American School Health Association. The National Adolescent Student Health Survey: A Report on the Health of America's Youth. Oakland, CA: Third Party Publishing Co, 1989.

12. Klepp KI, Perry CL, Jacobs DR. Etiology of drinking and driving among adolescents: implications for primary prevention. Health Educ Q 1991;18:415–427.

13. Williams AF, Lund AK, Preusser DF. Drinking and driving among high school students. Inter J Addict 1986;21:643–655.

14. Preusser D, Williams A, Zador P. The effect of curfew laws on motor vehicle crashes. Law Pol 1984;6:115–128.

15. Alexander E, Kallail K, Burdsal J, Ege D. Multifactorial causes of adolescent driver accidents: investigation of time as a major variable. J Adolesc Health Care 1990;11:413–417.

16. Robertson L, Zador P. Driver education and fatal crash involvement of teenaged drivers. Am J Public Health 1978;68:959–965.

17. Centers for Disease Control. Safety-belt and helmet use among high school students—United States, 1990. MMWR 1992;41:111–114.

18. National Highway Traffic Safety Administration. Restraint Use in 19 US Cities: 1989 Annual Report. Washington, DC: US Department of Transportation. DOT publication no. HS-807-595, 1990.

19. Rivara, F. Traumatic deaths of children in the United Sates: currently available prevention strategies. Pediatrics 1990;75:456–462.

20. Wasserman R, Waller J, Monty M, Emery A, Robinson D. Bicyclists, helmets, and head injuries: a rider-based study of helmet use and effectiveness. Am J Public Health 1988;78:1220–1221.

21. Cushman R, James W, Waclawik H. Physicians promoting bicycle helmets for children: a randomized trial. Am J Public Health 1991;81:1044–1046.

22. Logsdon DN, Lazaro CM, Meier RV. The feasibility of behavioral risk reduction in primary medical care. Am J Prev Med 1989;5:249–256.

23. Logsdon DN. Final Report of the INSURE Project. New York: Metropolitan Life, 1989.

24. Fingerhut LA, Kleinman JC, Godfrey E, Rosenberg H. Firearm mortality among children, youth, and young adults 1–34 years of age, trends and current status: United States, 1979–1988. Monthly Vital Statistics Report, National Center for Health Statistics, 39 (suppl), no. 11, 1991.

25. Fingerhut LA, Kleinman JC. Firearm mortality among children and youth. Adv Data 1989;178:1–6.

26. Christoffel KK, Christoffel T. Handguns as a pediatric problem. Pediatr Emerg Care 1986;2:75–81.

27. Wintemute GJ, Teret SP, Kraus JF, Wright M. The choice of weapons in firearm suicides. Am J Public Health 1988;78:824–826.

28. Christoffel KK. Toward reducing pediatric firearm injuries: charting a legislative and regulatory course. Pediatrics 1993 (in press).

29. Callahan CM, Rivara FP. Urban high school youth and handguns: a school-based survey. JAMA 1992;267:3038–3042.

30. Sadowski LS, Cairns RB, Earp JA. Firearm ownership among nonurban adolescents. Am J Dis Child 1989;143:1410–1413.

31. Runyan CW, Gerken EA: Epidemiology and prevention of adolescent injury: a review and research agenda. JAMA 1989;262:2273–2279.

32. Brent DA, Perper JA, Allman CJ, Moritz GM, Wartella ME, Zelenak JP: The presence and accessibility of firearms in the homes of adolescent suicides: a case-control study. JAMA 1991;266:2989–2995.

33. Sloan JH, Kellerman AL, Reahy DT, et al. Handgun regulations, crimes, assaults, and homicides: a tale of two cities. N Engl J Med 1990;319:1256–1262.

34. Sloan JH, Rivara FP, Reahy DT, et al. Firearm regulations and rates of suicide: a comparison of two metropolitan areas. N Engl J Med 1990;322:369–373.

35. Webster DW, Wilson MEH, Duggan AK, Pakula LC. Firearm injury prevention counseling: a study of pediatricians' beliefs and practices. Pediatrics 1992;89:902–907.

36. Webster DW, Wilson MEH, Duggan AK, Pakula LC. Parents' beliefs about preventing gun injuries to children. Pediatrics 1992;89:908–914.

37. Committee on Sports Medicine. Sports Medicine: Health Care for Young Athletes. Elk Grove, IL: American Academy of Pediatrics, 1983.

38. Garrick JG, Requa RK. Injuries in high school sports. Pediatrics 1978;61:465–469.

39. McLain LG, Reynolds S. Sports injuries in a high school. Pediatrics 1989;84:446–450.

40. Lysens R, Steverlynck A, van den Auweele Y. The predictability of sports injuries. Sports Med 1984;1:6–10.

41. Board of Trustees Report. Athletic Preparticipation Examinations for Adolescents. Chicago: American Medical Association, 1990.

42. Bradstock M, Marks J, Forman M, et al. Drinking-driving and health lifestyle in the United States: behavioral risk factors surveys. J Stud Alcohol 1987;48:147–152.

43. Wilson R. The relationship of seat belt use to personality, lifestyle and driving record. Health Ed Res 1990;5:175–185.

CHAPTER 5

Rationale and Recommendations: Dietary Habits, Eating Disorders, and Obesity

PREVENTION STRATEGY

GAPS recommends a strategy for the promotion of healthy dietary habits and the early identification of eating disorders and obesity. This strategy involves (1) providing health counseling to all adolescents annually about the benefits of proper diet, ways to achieve a healthy diet, and suggestions for safe weight management and (2) assessing weight and stature on all adolescents annually and asking adolescents annually about their body image and dieting patterns. Adolescents should be assessed for obesity (i.e., excessive fatness) if they have a Body Mass Index (BMI, weight per stature^2) equal to or greater than the 95% for gender and age, or if they gained two or more BMI points from the previous year. The determination of obesity is done by measuring skin fold thickness. Adolescents with a BMI between the 85th and 94th percentile are at risk for overweight and should be evaluated for factors associated with premature cardiovascular disease. In addition, they should be given general diet information and annual follow-ups. Obesity and low levels of activity are often complimentary conditions that should be addressed together.

Adolescents who have lost 10% of their previous weight, who have a BMI at the 5th percentile or less, who report inappropriate feelings of being overweight, or who use extreme measures to lose weight should be further assessed for the presence of anorexia nervosa or bulimia. These adolescents should also be evaluated to ensure they do not have an underlying organic disease that explains their condition. Physician guidelines for routine health guidance to promote healthy dietary habits and for the early identification of obesity, anorexia nervosa, and bulimia are included in GAPS Recommendations 7 and 13.

41

DISCUSSION

The busy lifestyle of today's families often results in adolescents skipping meals or relying on snack foods for basic nutrition. Survey results indicate that 34% of 8th grade and 45% of 10th grade students eat breakfast fewer than three days a week (1). Almost half of this population reports eating an average of three snacks a day; 60% of this food is high in fat or low in nutritional quality. The rapid physical growth of adolescence, however, requires a well-balanced diet to ensure adequate supplies of necessary nutrients. Low intakes of iron and calcium are of particular concern.

As few as 40% of adolescent males and 15% of adolescent females meet the dietary allowance for calcium (2). Failure to meet daily requirements for calcium may result in lowered bone mineral content which, in turn, may contribute to childhood fractures and osteoporosis in later life (3–5). Chan and associates noted higher bone mineral content and decreased risk of accidental fractures in children who consumed at least 60% of the daily recommended levels of calcium (4). In a retrospective study of women who were 49 to 66 years old, Sandler and associates found that regular consumption of dairy products during adolescence was associated with lower levels of postmenopausal bone loss (5). Inadequate calcium intake also appears to be associated with bone demineralization among lactating adolescent mothers, a process that is reversed with a high calcium diet (6).

Iron deficiency, which is predominantly related to inadequate dietary intake, is also relatively common among adolescents. Results of a national household survey (NHANES II) indicate that approximately 6% of females 11–14 years old and 14% of females 15–19 have low iron stores (7). Comparable figures for males are 12% for ages 11–14 and less than 1% for ages 15–19. Anemia, which occurs as a late stage of iron deficiency, is noted among 5% of males age 11–14 and approximately 2.5% of females age 11–19. Less than 1% of older adolescent males are anemic.

Adolescent athletes appear to have a higher prevalence of iron deficiency and associated anemia than do other adolescents (8–11). Strenuous exercise associated with endurance events may lower iron stores by causing chronic urinary or gastrointestinal blood loss and intravascular hemolysis (8, 9, 12). Results from an increasing number of studies are suggesting that iron deficiency, with associated anemia, has clinical significance for asymptomatic adolescents. Among athletes, anemia has been shown to decrease exercise capacity by diminishing maximum oxygen consumption, thus lowering endurance (8, 13). Other data suggest that iron deficiency anemia has an adverse affect on cognitive function (14–17). Iron supplementation has been shown, in some studies, to improve endurance and cognitive functioning (13–15).

In addition to diets that are frequently deficient in calcium and iron, many adolescents also consume excessive amounts of sodium and saturated fat. For example, data from the CDC Youth Risk Behavior Survey revealed that 27% of high school females and 43% of high school males eat more than two servings of food a day that are high in fat content (18). In another survey, 40% of 8th and 10th grade adolescents reported that they ate fast foods two or more times during the previous week, and 16% stated that they regularly added "a lot of salt" to their food (1). These dietary patterns can result in poor intake of other more nutritious foods, and they can lead to dietary problems during adolescence. They also contribute to establishing dietary habits and attitudes that may lead to health problems later in life.

Eating habits and attitudes influence not only the quality of the diet, but also an adolescent's emotional health. Disordered eating behaviors, including preoccupation with weight and use of extreme measures (e.g., diuretics, starvation, purging, and excessive exercise) to lose weight are common among adolescents. For example, a study of 8th and 10th grade students revealed that 3% of males and 11% of females used diet pills or candies to control weight; 2.5% of males and 7.5% of females reported that they control weight by vomiting after eating; almost 2.5% of males and 4% of females used laxatives to control weight; and 12% of males and 32.5% of females fasted (1). Overall, almost 5% of all males and 20% of females in the study had dieted four or more times during the previous year. Taken to an extreme, these behaviors suggest an emotional disturbance associated with anorexia nervosa or bulimia.

In a contemporary society that emphasizes thinness, many emotionally healthy adolescents exhibit some signs associated with pathological eating disorders. For instance, in a study of 326 adolescents, Moses and associates found that 51% of underweight high school females were fearful of obesity and 36% were preoccupied with body fat (19). Concern and preoccupation with thinness appear related to socioeconomic status (SES), race, and ethnicity. Using data from the National Health Examination Survey, Dornbush and associates reported that among adolescents age 12–17, females from higher SES family backgrounds had a greater desire for thinness than did females from families who were less advantaged economically (20). This relationship was consistent across levels of weight, but was not found for males. Data from the CDC Youth Risk Behavior Survey suggest that white and Hispanic females more frequently perceive themselves as overweight than do black females (18). In a study of high school students reported by

Story and associates, chronic dieting was reported by 8% of black females, 10.5% of Asian females, 11% of Native American females, 12.5% of white females, and 15% of Hispanic females (21). In summary, many adolescent have dietary habits that provide inadequate nutrients for physical growth and development. Adolescents are frequently concerned about their appearance and many use extreme measures to lose weight. The following sections will describe the frequency and health consequences of eating disorders (anorexia nervosa and bulimia) and obesity.

ANOREXIA NERVOSA AND BULIMIA

Anorexia nervosa and bulimia usually begin during adolescence. Anorexia nervosa is less common than bulimia and tends to start in somewhat younger adolescents. A variety of investigators have reported bulimia rates ranging from 2–20% for females and 1–5% for males (22, 23). This wide range in estimates reflects variation in the populations surveyed and inconsistency in criteria used to determine a psychiatric diagnosis. There is general consensus, however, that bulimia is found more frequently among white females from middle-class to upper-middle-class family backgrounds, and among adolescent athletes for whom weight control is a critical issue. Anorexia nervosa, which is also more common among white females, is estimated to occur in 1 in 200 adolescents (24).

Anorexia nervosa and bulimia are psychiatric disorders that tend to run extended courses lasting several years and resulting in severe physical, emotional, and behavioral consequences (25–27). The unique and striking characteristic of eating disorders is the adolescent's unrealistic, relentless pursuit of thinness. Regardless of how thin these adolescents might be, they are dissatisfied with the way they look and are obsessed with losing more weight. Various means are used to control weight, including excessive exercise, purging, diuretics, laxatives, and extreme dieting. Bingeing large quantities of food, followed by purging, are the hallmarks of bulimia. Adolescents with anorexia nervosa sometimes exhibit bingeing and purging behavior. Starvation, use of laxatives and diuretics, and recurrent vomiting often lead to sodium and potassium abnormalities. Hypokalemia and excessive use of ipecac adversely affect cardiac function and can lead to sudden death. The mortality rate from eating disorders is approximately 10%. Death can occur from the cardiotoxic effect of ipecac abuse, metabolic abnormalities (e.g., cardiac arrhythmias from hypokalemia), and suicide. A chronically inadequate diet, excessive use of measures to lose weight, and severe weight loss may also cause loss of bone mineral density, erosion of the dental enamel, esophageal hemorrhage, renal dysfunction, and chronic menstrual dysfunction (25–27).

OBESITY

Adolescence is a time of rapid changes in body size and composition. Before puberty, males and females have similar proportions of fat (approximately 15% and 19%, respectively), muscle, and lean body mass (28). During puberty, adolescent linear growth increases until it reaches the rate of 2-year-old children. For female adolescents, the percent of body fat increases to approximately 23% by age 20, while the percent of body fat for males decreases to approximately 12% by age 20. Because of these rapid changes, assessment of body composition, degree of adiposity, and obesity are more complicated for adolescents than for younger children or adults.

Data from a national sample of children suggest that among adolescents age 12–17, approximately 20% of white males, 13% of black males, 26% of white females, and 25% of black females are obese, where obesity is defined as a skin fold thickness greater than the 84th percentile for age (29). Excessive obesity, defined as a skin fold thicknesses greater than the 94th percentile, is found in 8%, 5%, 11%, and 12% of each of the four groups, respectively. Data from national surveys indicate that adolescent obesity is increasing, especially among black youth (29).

Obesity during adolescence has limited immediate physical or emotional implications. Obese adolescents do have somewhat higher blood pressure and may suffer from low self-esteem and depression (30–32). Although some obese adolescents demonstrate psychological differences from non-obese adolescents, these findings are not consistent and tend to vary with age and gender (33, 34). The major health problem associated with adolescent obesity is its relationship to risk of cardiovascular disease later in life. This relationship is based on two lines of evidence, one linking early onset obesity with adult obesity which, in turn, is associated with adult morbidity, and the other linking early onset obesity directly with increased adult morbidity.

Results of numerous studies provide strong evidence that the level of adiposity during infancy tracks into adolescence and that adolescent obesity continues into adulthood. Zack and associates, using data from two cycles of the Health Examination Survey, concluded that body fatness is a persistent characteristic from childhood into adolescence (35). Approximately 75% of children classified as obese remained obese when measured three to four years later. This relationship was independent of height, bone age, sexual maturation, or socioeconomic status.

In a study of urban black males, Johnston and Mack concluded that the risk ratio of obesity during adolescence was approximately 1.6 for children who had a high relative weight at the age of one (36). Charney and associates, in a retrospective study of 20–30-year-old adults, concluded that an individuals' weight in the first six months of life has a positive association to his or her weight during the third decade of life (37). In this study, 36% of infants exceeding the 90th percentile were overweight as adults, compared to 14% of average and light weight infants. Garn and LaVelle found that it is 1.77 times more likely that people who are obese as children will remain obese two decades later (38). Results from several longitudinal studies also support the continuity between early onset obesity and adult obesity (39–41). The findings in these studies demonstrate that, although not all young children and adolescents who are overweight become overweight adults, there is certainly a strong tendency for obesity to persist into adulthood. Interrupting this link has important implications for the prevention of adult morbidity and premature mortality.

Information from various studies demonstrates that adult obesity is an independent predictor of many disorders. These include, cardiovascular disease, hypertension, hypercholesterolemia, diabetes mellitus, gallbladder disease, arthritis, and gout (42–45). Adult obesity is also associated with a shorter life expectancy.

Evidence of a direct link between adolescent obesity and adult morbidity and mortality has been recently shown by Must and associates (46). Using longitudinal data from the Harvard Growth Study, these investigators found that males who were overweight at age 13–18 had an increased risk of mortality five to six decades later, compared to subjects who were lean during adolescence. Must and associates also found that both males and females who were overweight during adolescence were at greater risk for later cardiovascular disease and other morbidities. All of these risks were independent of adult weight.

JUSTIFICATION

Can Health Guidance Improve Diet Behaviors of Adolescents?

Evidence supporting the effectiveness of health guidance to improve diet is mainly provided from results of community and school-based studies on cardiovascular risk reduction. Perry and associates, in a study of 300 high school students, found that a health education program, providing social skills training on how to maintain a proper diet, increased knowledge and attitudes about healthy food choices (47). In another intervention to modify risks for cardiovascular disease, Killen and associates provided health education training to approximately 1,500 10th graders (48). Included in the intervention were special modules on nutrition and physical activity. Results obtained 12 months after the intervention indicated that the treatment group was significantly more likely than the control group to choose "heart healthy" food alternatives. In another study, Walter and associates investigated a school-based intervention directed at promoting healthy diet, exercise, and smoking prevention among approximately 3,400 children in New York (49). After five years, improvements were noted in level of serum cholesterol, quality of dietary intake, and knowledge about healthy dietary habits.

Expert opinion also supports the use and efficacy of dietary counseling for adolescents. In a recent report, the Expert Panel on Blood Cholesterol Levels in Children and Adolescents recommended that all youth be counseled to improve dietary habits in order to lower their average blood cholesterol (50). The objectives of this primary prevention strategy are to lower dietary saturated fatty acids, total fat, and cholesterol.

How Should Primary Care Physicians Assess Adolescents for Early Stages of Anorexia Nervosa or Bulimia?

Identification of adolescents with late stages of anorexia nervosa and bulimia is relatively straightforward. More challenging, however, is identifying adolescents who are in early stages of these diseases and appear outwardly healthy. Asking adolescents about their dieting patterns and satisfaction with their weight, and following weight and BMI, provide information that can be used to screen adolescents for early signs of eating disorders.

Early clinical signs of an eating disorder include unexplained weight loss and secondary amenorrhea. Anorexia nervosa should be considered in adolescents who have a drop in their BMI of two or more points. Metabolic changes, such as hypotension, hypothermia, and bradycardia occur with weight loss greater than 25% of ideal body weight and are, therefore, clinical signs found in more extreme situations (25, 27). Adolescents with this degree of weight loss are at medical risk for sudden death and should be treated as a medical emergency.

Chronic or extreme dieting behaviors are highly associated with dissatisfaction with weight. Moore found that 12–23-year-old females who were dissatisfied with their weight were more than twice as likely as other adolescents to fast; they were more than four times as likely to induce vomiting; and they were six times as likely to use stimulants (51). Dissatisfaction with body weight was reported by 53% of normal weight students and 40% of underweight students.

In another study, Story and associates investigated whether history of chronic dieting could be used to screen for anorexia nervosa or bulimia (21). Adolescents were classified as chronic dieters if they reported dieting continuously or if they had dieted 10 or more times during the previous year. Over 34,000 students from Minnesota public schools were surveyed and chronic dieting behavior was found for 12% of females and 2.1% of males. These rates varied from a low of 1.6% for 7th and 8th grade males to 14.3% for 11th and 12th grade females. Chronic dieters, compared to other adolescents, were 3 to 4 times more likely to report binge eating and fear of uncontrolled eating, and from 7 to 11 times more likely to report use of weekly self-induced vomiting, laxatives, diuretics, or ipecac to lose weight.

Results of the previous studies support the concept that, although most adolescents who report chronic dieting behaviors do not have anorexia nervosa or bulimia, the combination of these behaviors and a poor body image in an adolescent should alert the physician to perform a more in-depth assessment (21, 51). Several standardized questionnaires have been developed to assist in this evaluation. Probably the most widely used instruments are the Eating Attitudes Test (EAT) and the Eating Disorder Inventory. Both tests have been used extensively with adolescents and appear helpful in confirming a presumptive diagnosis of anorexia nervosa and bulimia (52).

The definitive diagnosis of anorexia nervosa or bulimia is made using standard psychiatric criteria (53). The diagnostic criteria for anorexia nervosa are:

- Refusal to maintain body weight over a minimum normal weight for age and height;
- Intense fear of gaining weight or becoming fat, even though underweight;
- Disturbance of body image—although underweight, the adolescent feels fat;
- In females, amenorrhea for at least three menstrual cycles.

The diagnostic criteria for bulimia include:

- Recurrent episodes of binge eating, defined as rapid consumption of large amounts of food during a short period of time;
- A feeling of lack of control during a binge;

- Use of self-induced vomiting, laxatives, diuretics, or other extreme means to prevent weight gain;
- A minimum of two binge episodes per week for at least three months;
- Persistent, excessive concern with body image.

How Effective is the Treatment for Anorexia Nervosa and Bulimia?

Depending on the severity of the initial symptoms, 33–86% of adolescents with anorexia nervosa have a satisfactory outcome (54–58). In a review of 12 major outcome studies, Schwartz and Thompson found that 6% of youth with anorexia nervosa had died, 38% were "cured," 23% improved, 14% had no marked improvement, and 26% had psychiatric impairment not related to anorexia nervosa (56). Herzog, in another review of outcome studies of patients with anorexia nervosa, also found wide variability in long-term treatment results (58). There was some indication that early identification and treatment led to more favorable outcomes.

Treatment for anorexia and bulimia usually includes psychotherapy, behavioral and family therapy, and nutritional education (56, 59, 60). Behavioral therapy may be successful during initial inpatient treatment, especially if it is individualized and developmentally oriented, and includes cognitive restructuring, education about weight and shape, and relapse prevention efforts (59). Fairburn and associates found significant improvements in dietary restraint, self-induced vomiting, attitude about weight, and EAT measures among patients who had received cognitive behavioral therapy as opposed to those who received either traditional interpersonal psychotherapy or behavioral therapy (59). Outcome studies and evaluation of treatment modalities of adolescents with bulimia, however, have not been as well studied as those for anorexia nervosa. Promising outcomes have been found with the use of antidepressant medications and with group therapy: 40–50% of patients show remission of symptoms with either modality (61).

The natural history of these disorders is often progressive emotional and physical disability, which may lead to death unless intervention occurs. Recommendations for screening for eating disorders, therefore, are substantiated by both a strong burden of suffering and scientific evidence on the need for early detection and treatment.

How Should Primary Care Physicians Assess Adolescents for Obesity?

Degree of body fat (i.e., obesity) is assessed in the clinical setting through measurements of body composition. This is usually done by obtaining anthropometric parameters, such as height, weight, or skin fold thickness. Skin fold thickness is considered the standard against which other clinical assessments of obesity are measured. Because of the complexities of measuring skin folds, however, most experts recommend that physicians use a relative weight/height scale to screen for overweight (62, 63). The results of various studies demonstrate a relatively high correlation between skin fold measurements and the body mass index, defined as weight/stature^2 (62–64). BMI varies with physical development, increasing in value from late childhood until the end of the pubertal growth spurt (63). Because no special equipment or time-consuming training is needed for reliable measurements, as is required for skinfold measurements, the BMI is recommended by GAPS to screen for overweight. It should be remembered, however, that extremes of height or lean tissue, such as may be seen with athletes, may distort findings. Once a presumptive diagnosis of obesity is made, the measurement of skin fold thickness can then be used to confirm that the adolescent has excessive body fat.

The guidelines for screening weight and stature were developed with the assistance of an expert panel convened by the AMA and the National Center for Education in Maternal Child Health to develop criteria specific for adolescents. This group of experts recommended using the BMI to screen for weight and stature and also recommended the assessment protocol used by GAPS (65). The BMI cut-off points by age for males and females are presented in the following two figures.

Interventions for treating adolescent obesity include developing a behavior modification plan for decreasing caloric intake and increasing exercise. Although no one method appears clearly better than others, treatment for adolescent obesity can be effective. In general, adolescents in treatment programs experience greater weight loss than do adolescents in control groups (66–73). Study results also suggest that beneficial results persist (65–67). Treatment is especially effective when adolescents are involved in programs that incorporate social skills training, diet counseling, and exercise—and when they involve parents in the management program (32, 67, 70–73). Benefits from weight loss include improved self-esteem, reduced depression, lowered blood pressure, elevated high-density lipoproteins and reduced serum triglycerides (66–68, 71–73).

Clinical Application

All adolescents should be provided with health guidance to help them develop dietary habits that promote healthy eating patterns and choices of food. To be effective, this guidance must have relevance for each adolescent. Some adolescents may see value in modifying their eating habits because of

Figure 5.1. Body Mass Index (BMI) by Age: Male

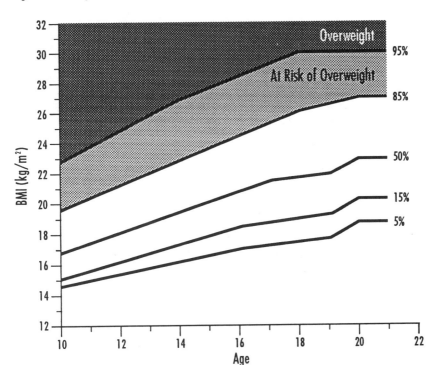

Source: Adopted from Himes J. H., Dietz W.H. Guidelines for Overweight in Adolescent Preventive Services. Chicago: American Medical Association, 1993.

a possible effect on athletic performance or on physical and emotional well-being. Others may be motivated by the possibility of losing or maintaining weight. The physician should find out what the adolescent sees as the benefit of dietary changes. The physician should then use this information to provide guidance, remaining sensitive to the fact that many adolescents, especially females, are concerned with their weight and body appearance.

GAPS recommends a two-step screening process for identifying adolescents who have anorexia nervosa and bulimia. Physicians can make a presumptive diagnosis of an eating disorder by identifying a constellation of emotional and behavioral changes, especially chronic dieting, extreme dissatisfaction with weight, low or declining BMI, or recent weight loss. A definitive diagnosis, however, requires a more detailed psychiatric and nutritional evaluation to determine emotional status, eating patterns, and

Figure 5.2. Body Mass Index (BMI) by Age: Female

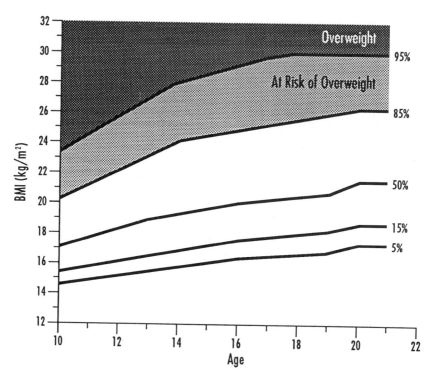

Source: Adopted from Himes J. H., Dietz W.H. Guidelines for Overweight in Adolescent Preventive Services.
Chicago: American Medical Association; 1993.

mechanisms used to control weight. Adolescents with signs of depressed metabolic status, such as hypothermia, hypotension, and bradycardia should have a careful physical evaluation, and hospitalization for medical management should be considered.

Although rare, other physical and psychiatric disorders may produce signs and symptoms that mimic anorexia nervosa or bulimia. These disorders include hypothyroidism, uncontrolled diabetes mellitus, occult malignancies, and severe depression. Adolescents with a suspected eating disorder should have a comprehensive medical evaluation to ensure their weight changes and anorexia do not have other causes.

The GAPS strategy also recommends that physicians use the BMI to screen adolescents for overweight. Because of the normal prepubertal accumulation of fat, care must be taken not to overdiagnose obesity. The recommendations presented in GAPS are conservative. Adolescents should be screened with the BMI; youths with a value equal to or greater than the 95th percentile for age and gender are considered overweight and need further assessment, including measurement of skin fold thickness. A diagnosis of obesity should only be made following the diagnostic assessment. The reason for this two-step approach is that some adolescents who are large and muscular may have high BMI values but not be obese (i.e., have excessive fat). Adolescents who are overweight should also be assessed for future risk for cardiovascular disease, including determining serum cholesterol (see Recommendation 12) and family history of hypertension, obesity, premature heart disease, and type I diabetes mellitus.

Adolescents between the 85th and 94th percentile are at risk for becoming overweight and should be followed annually. These adolescents should also be counseled about maintaining healthy diets and ensuring regular physical exercise.

REFERENCES

1. American School Health Association. The National Adolescent Student Health Survey: A Report on the Health of America's Youth. Oakland, CA: Third Party Publishing Co, 1989.

2. Morgan KJ, Stampley GL, Zabik ME, Fischer DR. Magnesium and calcium dietary intakes of the US population. J Am Coll Nutr 1985;4:195–206.

3. Chan GM. Dietary calcium and bone mineral status of children and adolescents. Am J Dis Child 1990;145:631–634.

4. Chan GM, Hess M, Hollis J, Book LS. Bone mineral status in childhood accidental injuries. Am J Dis Child 1984;138:569–570.

5. Sandler RB, Slemenda CW, LaPorte RE, et al. Post menopausal bone density and milk consumption in childhood and adolescence. Am J Clin Nutr 1985;42:270–274.

6. Chan GM, McMurray M, Westover K, Engelbert-Fenton K, Thomas MR. Effects of increased dietary calcium intake upon calcium and bone mineral status of lactating adolescent and adult women. Am J Clin Nutr 1987;46:319–323.

7. Expert Scientific Working Group (NHANES II). Report on the iron status in the US population assessed by NHANES II. Am J Clin Nutr 1985;42:1318–1330.

8. Raunklar RA, Sabio H. Anemia in the adolescent athlete. Am J Dis Child 1992;146:1201–1205.

9. Newhouse IJ, Clement DB. Iron status in athletes: an update. Sports Med 1988;5:337–352.

10. Nickerson HJ, Holubets M, Tripp AD, Pierce WE. Decreased iron stores in high school female runners. Am J Dis Child 1985;139:1115–1119.

11. Brown RT, McIntosh SM, Seabolt VR, Daniel WA. Iron status of adolescent female athletes. J Adolesc Health Care 1985;6:349–352.

12. Nickerson HJ, Holubets M, Weiler B, Haas R, Schwartz S, Ellefson M. Causes of iron deficiency in adolescent athletes. J Pediatr 1989;114:657–663.

13. Rowland TW, Deisroth MB, Green GM, Kelleher JF. The effect of iron therapy on the exercise capacity of nonanemic iron-deficient adolescent runners. Am J Dis Child 1988;142:165–169.

14. Pollitt E, Soemantri AG, Yunis F, Scrimshaw NS. Cognitive effects of iron deficiency anemia. Lancet 1985;1:158.

15. Soemantri AG, Pollitt E, Kim I. Iron deficiency anemia and educational achievement. Am J Clin Nutr 1985;42:1221–1228.

16. Groner JA, Holtzman NA, Charney E, Mellits ED. A randomized trial of oral iron on tests of short-term memory and attention span in young pregnant women. J Adolesc Health Care 1986;7:44–48.

17. Ballin A, Berar M, Rubinstein U, Kleter Y, Hershkovitz A, Meytes D: Iron state in female adolescents. Am J Dis Child 1992;146:803–805.

18. Centers for Disease Control. Body-weight perceptions and selected weight-management goals and practices of high school students: United States, 1990. MMWR 1991;40:741,747–750.

19. Moses N, Banilivy MM, Lifshitz F. Fear of obesity among adolescent girls. Pediatrics 1989;83:393–398.

20. Dornbush SM, Carlsmith JM, Duncan PD, et al. Sexual maturation, social class, and the desire to be thin among adolescent females. Dev Behav Pediatr 1984;5:308–314.

21. Story M, Rosenwinklel K, Himes JH, Resnick M, Harris LJ, Blum RW. Demographic and risk factors associated with chronic dieting in adolescents. Am J Dis Child 1991;145:994–998.

22. Conners ME, Johnson CL. Epidemiology of bulimia and bulimic behaviors. Addict Behav 1987;12:165–179.

23. Drewnowski A, Hopkins SA, Kessler RC. The prevalence of bulimia nervosa in the US college student population. Am J Public Health 1988;78:1322–1325.

24. Pope HG, Hudson JL, Yurgelun-Todd D, Hudson MS. Prevalence of anorexia nervosa and bulimia in three student populations. Int J Eat Disorders 1984;3:45–51.

25. Herzog DB, Copeland PM. Eating disorders. N Engl J Med 1985;313:295–303.

26. Bachrach LK, Guido D, Katzman D, Litt IF, Marcus R. Decreased bond density in adolescent girls with anorexia nervosa. Pediatrics 1990;86:440–447.

27. Palla B, Litt IF. Medical complications of eating disorders in adolescents. Pediatrics 1988;81:613–623.

28. Garn SM, Clark DC. Trends in fatness and the origins of obesity. Pediatrics 1976;57:443–455.

29. Gortmaker SL, Dietz WH, Sobol AM, Wehler CA. Increasing pediatric obesity in the United States. Am J Dis Child 1987;141:535–540.

30. Kaplan KM, Wadden TA. Childhood obesity and self-esteem. J Pediatr 1986;109:367–370.

31. Martin S, Housley K, McCoy H, et al. Self-esteem of adolescent girls as related to weight. Percept Mot Skills 1988;67:879–884.

32. Rocchini AP, Katch V, Anderson J, et al. Blood pressure in obese adolescents: effect of weight loss. Pediatrics 1988;82:16–23.

33. Klesges RC. Personality and obesity: global versus specific measures? Beh Assess 1984;6:347–356.

34. Mendelson BK, White DR. Development of self-body-esteem in overweight youngsters. Dev Psychol 1985;21:90–96.

35. Zack PM, Harlan WR, Leaverton PE, Cornoni-Huntley JC. A longitudinal study of body fatness in childhood and adolescence. J Pediatr 1979;95:126–130.

36. Johnston FE, Mack RW. Obesity in urban black adolescents of high and low relative weight at 1 year of age. Am J Dis Child 1978;132:862–864.

37. Charney E, Goodman HC, McBride M, Lyon B, Pratt R. Childhood antecedents of adult obesity: do chubby infants become obese adolescents? N Engl J Med 1976;295:6–9.

38. Garn SM, LaVelle M. Two-decade follow-up of fatness in early childhood. Am J Dis Child 1985;139:181–185.

39. Cronk CE, Roche AF, Kent R, et al. Longitudinal trends and continuity in weight/stature^2 from 3 months to 18 years. Hum Biol 1982;54:729–749.

40. Cronk CE, Roche AF, Chumlea WC, Kent R. Longitudinal trends of weight/stature^2 in childhood in relationship to adulthood body fat measures. Hum Biol 1982;54:751–764.

41. Siervogel RM, Roche AF, Guo S, Mukherjee D, Chumlea WC. Patterns of change in weight/stature^2 from 2 to 18 years: findings from long-term serial data for children in the Fels longitudinal growth study. Int J Obes 1991; 15:479–485.

42. Hubert H, Feinleib M, McNamara PM, Castelli WP. Obesity as an independent risk factor for cardiovascular disease: a 26-year follow-up of participants in the Framingham Heart Study. Circulation 1983;67:968–977.

43. Burton BT, Foster WR, Hirsch J, Van Itallie TB. Health implications of obesity: an NIH consensus development conference. Int J Obes 1985;9:155–169.

44. Van Itallie TB. Health implications of overweight and obesity in the United States. Ann Intern Med 1985;103:983–988.

45. Simopoulos AP, Van Itallie TB. Body weight, health, and longevity. Ann Intern Med 1984;100:285–295.

46. Must A, Jacques PF, Dallal GE, Bajema CJ, Dietz WH. Long-term morbidity and mortality of overweight adolescents: a follow-up of the Harvard Growth Study of 1922 to 1935. N Engl J Med 1992;327:1350–1355.

47. Perry CL, Klepp KI, Halper A, et al. Promoting healthy eating and physical activity patterns among adolescents: a pilot study of "slice of life." Health Ed Res 1987;2:93–103.

48. Killen JD, Telch MJ, Robinson TN, Maccoby N, Taylor CB, Farquhar JW. Cardiovascular risk reduction for tenth graders. JAMA 1988;260:1728–1733.

49. Walter H, Hofman A, Vaughan R, Wynder E. Modification of risk factors for coronary heart disease: five-year results of a school-based intervention trial. N Engl J Med 1988;318:1093–1100.

50. Expert Panel on Blood Cholesterol Levels in Children and Adolescents. National cholesterol education program. Pediatrics 1992;89(Part 2):525–584.

51. Moore DC. Body image and eating behavior in adolescent girls. Am J Dis Child 1988;142:1114–1118.

52. Williams RL. Use of the Eating Attitudes Test and Eating Disorder Inventory in adolescents. J Adolesc Health Care 1987;8:266–272.

53. American Psychiatric Association. Diagnostic and Statistical Manual of Mental Disorders (3rd edition revised). Washington, DC: American Psychiatric Association, 1987.

54. Kreipe RE, Churchill BH, Strauss J. Long-term outcome of adolescents with anorexia nervosa. Am J Dis Child 1989;143:1322–1327.

55. Nussbaum M, Shenker RI, Baird D, Saravay S. Follow-up investigation in patients with anorexia nervosa. J Pediatr 1985;106:835–840.

56. Schwartz DM, Thompson MG. Do anorectics get well? Current research and future needs. Am J Psychiatry 1981;138:319–323.

57. Hsu LKG, Crisp AH. Outcome of anorexia nervosa. Lancet 1979;8107:61–65.

58. Herzog DB, Keller MB, Lavori PW. Outcome in anorexia nervosa and bulimia nervosa. J Nerv Ment Dis 1988;176:131–143.

59. Fairburn CG, Jones R, Peveler RC, et al. Three psychological treatments for bulimia nervosa. Arch Gen Psychiatry 1991;48:463–469.

60. Liebman R, Sargent J, Silver M. A family systems orientation to the treatment of anorexia nervosa. J Am Acad Child Adolesc Psychiatry 1983;22:128–133.

61. Pope HG, Hudson JI, Jonas JM, Yurgelun-Todd D. Antidepressant treatment of bulimia: a two-year follow-up study. J Clin Psychopharmacol 1985;5:320–327.

62. Himes JH, Bouchard C. Validity of anthropometry in classifying youths as obese. Int J Obes 1989;13:183–193.

63. Cole TJ. Weight-stature indices to measure underweight, overweight, and obesity. In: Himes JH, ed. Anthropometric Assessment of Nutritional Status. New York: John Wiley & Sons, 1991:83–111.

64. Michielutte R, Diseker RA, Corbett WT, Schey HM, Ureda JR. The relationship between weight-height indices and the triceps skinfold measure among children age 5 to 12. Am J Public Health 1984;74:604–606.

65. Himes JH, Dietz WH. Guidelines for overweight in adolescent preventive services: recommendations from the Expert Committee on Clinical Guidelines for Overweight in Adolescent Preventive Services. (In preparation).

66. Becque M, Katch VL, Rocchini A, Marks CR, Moorehead C. Coronary risk incidence of obese adolescents: reduction by exercise plus diet intervention. Pediatrics 1988; 81:605–612.

67. Epstein LH, Kuller LH, Wing RR, Valoski A, McCurley J. The effect of weight control on lipid changes in obese children. Am J Dis Child 1989;143:454–457.
68. Mellin LM, Slinkard LA, Irwin CE. Validation of the SHAPEDOWN adolescent obesity intervention. J Am Diet Ass 1987;87:333–338.
69. Epstein LH, Valoski A, Wing RR, McCurley J. Ten-year follow-up of behavioral family-based treatment for obese children. JAMA 1990;264:2519–2523.
70. Epstein LH, Wing RR, Penner BC, Kress MJ. Effect of diet and controlled exercise on weight loss in obese children. J Pediatr 1985;107:358–361.
71. Coates TJ, Killen JD, Slinkard LA. Parent participation in a treatment program for overweight adolescents. Int J Eat Disorders 1982;1:37–47.
72. Brownell KD, Kelman JH, Stunkard AJ. Treatment of obese children with and without their mothers: changes in weight and blood pressure. Pediatrics 1983;71:515–523.
73. Wadden TA, Stunkard AJ, Rich L, Rubin CJ, Sweidel G, McKinney S. Obesity in black adolescent girls: a controlled clinical trial of treatment by diet, behavioral modification, and parental support. Pediatrics 1990;85:345–352.

CHAPTER 6

Rationale and Recommendation: Physical Fitness

PREVENTION STRATEGY

GAPS recommends that physicians provide health guidance on an annual basis to all adolescents in order to promote improved physical fitness. This should include health guidance about the emotional, social, and physical benefits of exercise and encouragement to exercise regularly. Physician guidelines for fitness are addressed by GAPS Recommendation 8.

DISCUSSION

Physical activity can be defined as ". . . any body movement produced by skeletal muscles that results in energy expenditure" (1). There are various types of physical activity, including exercise, such as participation in organized sports and aerobic conditioning; household tasks, such as performing yard work and home repairs; and other leisure time activities, such as unorganized, recreational activities (1–3). The greatest emotional and physiological benefit appears to result from physical exercise, which can be defined as ". . . activity that is planned, structured, repetitive, and purposeful in the sense that improvement or maintenance of one or more components of physical activity is the objective" (2).

Physical fitness is commonly viewed as a personal attribute that people achieve from regular physical activity (i.e., exercise). During the past several decades, the definition of fitness has evolved, with a change in focus from "motor fitness," which includes factors such as strength and speed, to "health-related fitness," which includes cardiovascular endurance, body composition, flexibility, and muscular strength and endurance (1–3). This later concept directs attention at the value of fitness for improving not only the ability of a person to accomplish work, but also the benefits associated with lower risk for cardiovascular disease, improved psychological status, and reduced risk of musculoskeletal disorders. Since it is usually correlated with fitness, physical activity is often used as a proxy measure for fitness because it is easy to assess and can serve as a basis for health counseling.

In one of the few national studies assessing the physical activity level of children, data from the 1984 and 1986 National Children and Youth Fitness Study suggest that approximately 66% of children in grades 5–12 engage in regular aerobic exercise performed at least three times a week for at least 20 minutes a session (4, 5).

Another measure of level of physical activity is the frequency of participation and quality of exercise provided in school physical education (PE) classes. National data on adolescents' involvement in PE are provided by the CDC's Youth Risk Behavior Surveillance System. Data from 1990 indicated that 57% of high school females and 48% of high school males were enrolled in PE classes (6). Enrollment, however, declined substantially between the 9th and 12th grades. Of those who attended PE classes during the previous two weeks, only 33% exercised at least three times a week for 20 minutes and 23% reported that they did not exercise at all. When asked if they had exercised vigorously, only 37% reported they did so three or more times a week (7).

Exercise, whether moderate or vigorous, was reported less by females, black students, and students in the higher grades. An inverse relation between watching TV or videos and vigorous exercise was noted for females, but not for males. These data suggest that while participation in PE classes provides an opportunity for regular exercise, the majority of a youth's physical exercise occurs outside of school. This conclusion is supported by results from the Children and Youth Fitness Study. Although 52% of students participated in PE classes three or more times a week, over 80% of a youth's average weekly physical activity occurred outside of school (4, 5).

Estimates of the level of physical fitness among children and youth come predominantly from studies on the effect of cardiovascular risk reduction programs. Zuckerman and associates studied risk factors for future cardiovascular disease among 4th to 6th grade students enrolled in four Know Your Body Programs around the country (8). The level of cardiovascular physical fitness was assessed using a modified version of the Harvard step test. Overall, black students were more likely to be physically fit (rates of 60–88%) than were white or Hispanic children (rates of 54–82%). Data from one of the programs indicated that more males than females were fit (71% vs. 51%). In a smaller study, again using the modified Harvard step test, Desmond and associates found that 60–70% of 257 adolescents had average-to-good physical fitness (9). Although there were no racial differences in rates of fitness, a strong relationship between reported exercise practices and physical fitness was noted for black, but not white, students. The results of these studies and others suggest that, compared to adults, the level of physical activity and fitness among children and adolescents is relatively high (10).

JUSTIFICATION

Do Fitness Behaviors Developed During Adolescence Track into Adulthood?

Although the level of physical activity and physical fitness among children and adolescents is relatively high, these parameters decline throughout the life span. Stephens and associates analyzed the epidemiology of leisure-time physical activity using results from eight national surveys of adults conducted in the United States and Canada and concluded that: (1) younger people participate more frequently in "active" leisure-time physical activity than do adults and older people, (2) the steepest decline in physical activity occurs between mid-childhood and adolescence; although less participation in sports is a factor, this decline is also related to a reduction in leisure time activity, and (3) males and individuals from upper income groups are more physically active than are females and people from families with less income (11).

There is moderate support, however, for a positive relationship between a person's level of physical activity and fitness during adolescence and this level as an adult. Dishman and associates reviewed determinants of adult physical activity and exercise, and found that participation as a youth in organized sports (but not necessarily informal recreational activities) was associated with engaging in vigorous physical activity as an adult (12). A stronger association was found for females and for youths who participated in more than one sport. The authors concluded ". . . that while exercise or sport experience in youth can be a strong agent in influencing exercise behavior in adults, its influence is frequently overridden by other personal and environmental influences."

In another study, Dennison and associates compared the physical activity levels of 453 young men 23–25 years old with their physical fitness scores as children (13). Responses to questions about their current level of activity were used to determine a score reflecting their average work intensity. Based on this figure, subjects were divided into a physically active group (65% of subjects) and an inactive group (35% of subjects). When compared to the inactive group, adults in the active group had significantly better standardized fitness test scores as children. This group also participated in more organized sports since high school, had greater parental encouragement for sports as a child, and had greater encouragement for exercise by their spouse. In conflict with the studies previously discussed, however, Powell and Dysinger reviewed six prominent studies and determined that data were inconclusive in support of a relationship between participation in organized school sports or physical education as a child and physical activity level as an adult (14). Sallis and associates also found an insignificant relationship between vigorous physical activity level as an adult and a history of physical activity as an adolescent (15). In a recent review of studies published on this topic, Sallis and McKenzie conclude that "the most parsimonious conclusion from these studies is that the findings conflict" (16).

In summary, although there is some research support for the tracking of physical activity from childhood and adolescence to adulthood, data are conflicting. Reasons for this include: (1) the retrospective methodology most commonly utilized is better-suited to track past physical activities that are easily remembered, such as participation in vigorous or organized sports, rather than participation in other forms of more moderate types of physical activity, (2) many studies use vigorous exercise as the outcome measure, rather than more moderate forms of physical activity, and (3) intervening variables, such as changes in physical status and psychosocial factors, alter an adult's ability, opportunity, and enthusiasm for exercise.

Does a Greater Level of Physical Activity and Fitness Improve Health?

The most well-documented health effect of exercise and physical fitness is the association, among adults, between a sedentary lifestyle and risk factors for adult cardiovascular disease and premature death (17–24). The level of fitness influences heart disease both directly and indirectly through its effect on blood pressure, serum lipid levels, and obesity. Physical activity and fitness of adults also increase insulin sensitivity which, in turn, leads to improved diabetic control and, possibly, reduced risk of noninsulin-dependent diabetes mellitus. Finally, high levels of physical activity of adults has also been shown to reduce the rate of different kinds of cancer, osteoporosis, musculoskeletal injury, anxiety, and depression (25–30).

Although the scientific evidence is less robust, level of physical activity and fitness is also associated with cardiovascular risk factors among adolescents, including obesity, blood pressure, and lipid levels (31–36). This association appears unrelated to race or gender, but is partially related to weight and stature. Thus, children and adolescents who are heavier or larger obtain more cardiovascular benefit from increasing their physical activity than do other youth. An additional benefit of routine exercise for adolescents is reduced depression and improvement in emotional well-being (37–39). For example, Goldwater and Collis randomly assigned university students to aerobic (vigorous cardiovascular exercise) and non-aerobic (motor activities with minimal cardiovascular benefit) treatments (37). Students in the aerobic group had significantly greater improvement in cardiovascular fitness, greater reduction in anxiety, and increased emotional well-being compared to the other students.

There is uncertainty regarding the amount of physical activity needed to produce fitness, promote emotional health, and reduce morbidity and premature mortality. Current recommendations, however, are that children and adolescents engage in physical activity (preferably aerobic exercise) that requires movement of the large muscle groups at least three times a week for 20–30 minutes. The goal is to achieve moderate-intensity exertion, often defined as maintaining 75% of maximum heart rate (40). The dose-response relationship between physical activity and fitness, however, does not appear to be a dichotomous "all or nothing" phenomenon. In a review of studies investigating the relationship between levels of physical activity and morbidity and mortality, Blair and associates concluded that even moderate levels of activity are associated with beneficial effects in health (27).

Can Fitness Behaviors of Adolescents Be Improved Through Office Counseling?

Results from several office-based studies suggest that physician advice can increase level of physical activity in adults (41, 42). For example, Lewis and Lynch provided a brief preventive intervention to young adult patients who were seen in a family practice clinic (41). Data obtained at one month follow-up demonstrated that patients who had received the intervention, compared to control group patients, increased the duration but not the frequency of their physical exercise. Results from the INSURE Project (Industrywide Network for Social, Urban and Rural Efforts), also involved an office-based preventive intervention and demonstrated that physician health education can have a moderate influence on the initiation of physical activity in adults (42).

Results from various studies suggest that adolescent risk factors for future cardiovascular disease, including physical activity, can be improved through a school or community-based health education program (16, 43, 44). For example, Killen and associates found that a school-based cardiovascular risk reduction program directed at almost 1,500 10th grade students had a significant effect on the initiation of strenuous physical activity

(43). At the time of the baseline assessment, approximately 30% of both a treatment and a control group reported regular aerobic physical activity. Of these students, an additional 30% who received the health education intervention compared to 20% who were in the control group reported they were exercising regularly at the two month follow-up assessment. Results from other studies also suggest that the level of physical activity children engage in during school PE classes and outside of school can be increased by a targeted intervention (16, 44). Studies to date, however, have not attempted to promote exercise among adolescents from an office-based approach.

Additional support for this recommendation is provided by data from studies investigating factors associated with adolescent physical activity and fitness. Desmond and associates studied 257 high school students and found that, among white adolescents, seven psychosocial factors distinguished youths who had good physical fitness from those who did not (9). The strongest variables were "many of my friends regularly exercise"; "if my doctor told me to exercise I would do so"; and "if I do not exercise I will get out of shape." Among black adolescents, the two strongest variables that distinguished the physically fit from the nonfit group were "perceived fitness status" and "intention to be a regular exerciser five years from now."

Regardless of fitness status and race, 70–80% of adolescents reported that "if my doctor told me to exercise I would do so." Because of their credibility, the advice provided by physicians and other health professionals may have especially high relevance for adolescents. The results of other studies support the concept that the physical activity level of adolescents is influenced by their perception that involvement in exercise is something that people who are close to them believe they should do (45–47). Taken together, the results of the study by Desmond (in which physician influence was identified directly) and results of these later studies (which suggest a theoretical influence of health providers) imply that office-based support and encouragement might have a beneficial effect in promoting physical activity of adolescents.

CLINICAL APPLICATION

Health guidance to promote physical fitness should focus on the broad set of physical activities that adolescents can do to improve their level of fitness. Regular physical activity should become a component of a healthy lifestyle. Adolescents should be helped, therefore, to determine the most enjoyable form of activity for them, whether it be organized sports or recreational activities. They should be encouraged to develop physical activity habits they will be likely to continue. Physicians should counsel adolescents about the physiologic and psychologic benefits of exercise and work with each adolescent to develop a "prescription" for exercise. Compliance with this exercise regimen can be improved by (1) helping the adolescent identify the social factors that promote or inhibit their participation in regular physical activity, (2) using mutually agreed upon goals for exercise that are specific for the individual adolescent, and (3) advising adolescents that any regular physical activity, even brisk walks or recreational bicycle riding, is good for their health (3). Finally, adolescents should also be encouraged to participate in school physical education classes throughout secondary school and to use these classes as an opportunity to develop a habit of regular physical exercise.

REFERENCES

1. Caspersen CJ, Powell KE, Christenson GM. Physical activity, exercise, and physical fitness: definitions and distinctions for health-related research. Pub Health Rep 1985; 100:126–131.

2. Pate RR. A new definition of youth fitness. Phys Sports Med 1983;11:77–83.

3. Rauniker RA, Strong WB. The status of adolescent physical fitness. In: Dyment PG, ed. Adolescent Medicine: State of the Art Reviews (Vol. 2). Philadelphia: Hamnley and Belfus, 1991:65–77.

4. Ross JG, Gilbert GG. The National Children and Youth Fitness Study: a summary of findings. J Phys Ed Recr Dance 1985;56:45–50.

5. Ross JG, Pate RR. The National Children and Youth Fitness Study II: a summary of findings. J Phys Ed Recr Dance 1987;58:51–56.

6. Centers for Disease Control. Participation of high school students in school physical education: United States, 1990. MMWR 1991;40:613–615.

7. Centers for Disease Control. Vigorous physical activity among high school students: United States, 1990. MMWR 1992;41:33–35.

8. Zuckerman AE, Peleg EO, Bush PJ, et al. Cardiovascular risk factors among black schoolchildren: comparisons among four Know Your Body studies. Prev Med 1989;18:113–132.

9. Desmond SM, Price JH, Lock RS, Smith D, Stewart PW. Urban black and white adolescents' physical fitness status and perceptions of exercise. J Sch Health 1990;60:220–226.

10. Simons-Morton BG, O'Hara NM, Simons-Morton DG, Parcel GS. Children and fitness: a public health perspective. Res Q Exerc Sport 1987;58:295–302.

11. Stephens T, Jacobs DR, White CC. A descriptive epidemiology of leisure-time physical activity. Pub Health Reports 1985;100:147–157.

12. Dishman RK, Sallis JF, Orenstein DR. The determinants of physical activity and exercise. Pub Health Reports 1985;100:158–172.
13. Dennison BA, Straus JH, Mellits ED, Charney E. Child physical fitness tests: predictor of adult activity levels. Pediatrics 1988;82:324–330.
14. Powell KE, Dysinger W. Childhood participation in organized school sports and physical education as precursors of adult physical activity. Am J Prev Med 1987;3:276–281.
15. Sallis JF, Hovell MF, Hofstetter CR, et al. A multivariate study of determinants of vigorous exercise in a community sample. Prev Med 1989;18:20–34.
16. Sallis JF, McKenzie TL. Physical education's role in public health. Res Q Exerc Sport 1991;62:124–137.
17. Sallis JF, Haskell WL, Wood PD. Vigorous physical activity and cardiovascular risk factors in young adults. J Chronic Dis 1986;39:115–120.
18. Wood PD, Haskell WL, Blair SN. Increased exercise level and plasma lipoprotein concentrations: a one-year, randomized, control study in sedentary, middle-aged men. Metabolism 1983;32:31–39.
19. Paffenberger RS, Hyde RT. Exercise in the prevention of coronary heart disease. Prev Med 1984;13:3–22.
20. Leon AS, Connett J, Jacobs DR, Rauramaa R. Leisure-time physical activity levels and risk of coronary heart disease and death: the multiple risk factor intervention trial. JAMA 1987;258:2388–2395.
21. Paffenbarger RS, Hyde RT, Wing AL, Hsieh C. Physical activity, all-cause mortality, and longevity of college alumni. N Engl J Med 1986;314:605–613.
22. Blair SN, Kohl HW, Paffenbarger RS, Clark DG, Cooper KH, Gibbons LW. Physical fitness and all-cause mortality: a prospective study of healthy men and women. JAMA 1989;262:2395–2401.
23. Kannel WB, Wilson P, Blair SN. Epidemiological assessment of the role of physical activity and fitness in development of cardiovascular disease. Am Heart J 1985;109:876–885.
24. Wood PD, Stefanick ML, Dreon DM, et al. Changes in plasma lipids and lipoproteins in overweight men during weight loss through dieting as compared with exercise. N Engl J Med 1988;319:1173–1179.
25. Powell KE, Caspersen CJ, Koplan JP, Ford ES. Physical activity and chronic diseases. Am J Clin Nutr 1989;49:999–1006.
26. Stephens T. Physical activity and mental health in the United States and Canada: evidence from four population surveys. Prev Med 1988;17:35–47.
27. Blair SN, Kohl HW, Gordon NF, Paffenbarger RS. How much physical activity is good for health? Annu Rev Public Health 1992;13:99–126.
28. Recker RR, Davies M, Hinders SM, Heaney RP, Stegman MR, Kimmel DB. Bone gain in young adult women. JAMA 1992;268:2403–2408.
29. McCann IL, Holmes DS. Influence of aerobic exercise on depression. J Pers Soc Psychol 1984;46:1142–1147.
30. Rape R. Running and depression. Percept Mot Skills 1987;64:1303–1310.

31. Fraser GE, Phillips RL, Harris R. Physical fitness and blood pressure in children. Circulation 1983;67:405–412.

32. Fripp RR, Hodgson JL, Kwiterovitch PO, Werner JC, Schuler HG, Whitman V. Aerobic capacity, obesity, and atherosclerotic risk factors in male adolescents. Pediatrics 1985;75:813–818.

33. Sallis JF, Patterson TL, Buono MJ, Nader PR. Relation of cardiovascular fitness and physical activity to cardiovascular disease risk factors in children and adults. Am J Epidemiol 1988;127:933–941.

34. Durant RH, Linder CW, Mahoney, OM. Relationship between habitual physical activity and serum lipoprotein levels in white male adolescents. J Adolesc Health Care 1983;4:235–240.

35. Kuntzleman CT, Reiff GG. The decline in American children's fitness levels. Res Q Exerc Sport 1992;63:107–111.

36. Hagberg JM, Goldring D, Ehsani AA, et al. Effect of exercise training on the blood pressure and hemodynamic features of hypertensive adolescents. Am J Cardiol 1983;52:763–768.

37. Goldwater RC, Collis ML. Psychologic effects of cardiovascular conditioning: a controlled experiment. Psychosom Med 1985;47:174–181.

38. Brown JD, Lawton M. Stress and well-being in adolescence: the moderating role of physical exercise. J Hum Stress 1986;(Fall):125–131.

39. Collingwood TR, Reynolds R, Kohl HW, Smith W, Sloan S. Physical fitness effects on substance abuse risk factors and use patterns. J Drug Educ 1991;21:73–84.

40. Simons-Morton BG, Parcel GS, O'Hara NM, Blair SN, Pate RR. Health-related physical fitness in childhood: status and recommendations. Annu Rev Public Health 1988;9:403–425.

41. Lewis BS, Lynch WD. The effect of physician advice on exercise behavior. Prev Med 1993;22:110–121.

42. Logsdon DN, Lazaro CM, Meier RV. The feasibility of behavioral risk reduction in primary medical care. Am J Prev Med 1989;5:249–256.

43. Killen JD, Telch MJ, Robinson TN, Maccoby N, Taylor CB, Farquhar JW. Cardiovascular disease risk reduction for tenth graders. JAMA 1988;260:1728–1733.

44. Perry CL, Klepp KI, Halper A, et al. Promoting healthy eating and physical activity patterns among adolescents: a pilot study of "slice of life." Health Ed Res 1987;2:93–103.

45. Reynolds KD, Killen JD, Bryson SW, et al. Psychosocial predictors of physical activity in adolescents. Prev Med 1990;19:541–551.

46. Greennockle KM, Lee AA, Lomax R. The relationship between selected student characteristics and activity patterns in a required high school physical education class. Res Q Exerc Sport 1990;61:59–69.

47. Godin G, Shephard RJ. Psychosocial factors influencing intentions to exercise of young students from grades 7 to 9. Res Q Exerc Sport 1986;57:41–52.

CHAPTER 7

Rationale and Recommendations: Psychosexual Development and the Negative Health Consequences of Sexual Behaviors

PREVENTION STRATEGY

Learning to develop appropriate sexual attitudes and behaviors is a major component of adolescence. The health risks associated with HIV infection only accentuate the necessity for developing responsible sexual behavior. GAPS recommends a comprehensive primary and secondary prevention strategy for promoting healthy psychosexual development and preventing the negative consequences of sexual behaviors. This strategy includes: (1) providing health guidance to adolescents to promote a better understanding of psychosexual development—how HIV infection is transmitted, the dangers of the disease, the effectiveness of latex condoms in preventing STDs, including HIV infection; the dangers of coercive sexual practices; the effectiveness of sexual abstinence, the best way to prevent STD infection and pregnancy; information about contraceptive devices; (2) screening to identify adolescents who are engaging in sexual behaviors that might result in unintended pregnancy or STDs, including HIV infection; screening of sexually active adolescents for STDs, including gonorrhea, chlamydia, genital warts, and syphilis; offering HIV testing to adolescents who engage in high-risk sexual behaviors; and (3) immunizing selected adolescents against hepatitis B virus.

GAPS also advocates that physicians ensure latex condoms and other appropriate methods of birth control are available in their clinical setting to adolescents. Physicians should be especially aware of the association between unsafe sexual behavior and the use of alcohol and other drugs—identification of one behavior should lead the practitioner to search for the other. As with other sensitive topics, counseling and screening for sexual behaviors is best done in a confidential manner. Physician guidelines for health guidance for normal psychosexual development and sexual behaviors are addressed in GAPS Recommendations 5 and 9; screening for sexual behavior is addressed in GAPS Recommendation 16; screening for STDs and HIV infection are addressed in Recommendations 17 and 18; the guidelines for immunization against hepatitis B virus are contained in GAPS Recommendation 24.

DISCUSSION

"Initiating sexual activity is a natural transition made by nearly all humans. It is not the occurrence of this transition but its timing and the circumstances under which it occurs that can have significant implications" (1).

Trends over the past several decades suggest that more adolescents than ever before are engaging in sexual intercourse, are initiating sexual intercourse at earlier ages, and are having intercourse with more sexual partners (2–5). Over 50% of females and 60% of males between 15 and 19 years of age have had sexual intercourse (3). These figures represent an increase of 33% from just two decades ago (see Fig. 7.1). Similar trends are found for even younger adolescents: 18% of 15-year-old females and 28% of 16-year-old females are sexually active, representing increases of 24% and 34% respectively from the early 1970s. By the time they are seniors, 67% of females and 76% of males have had sexual intercourse (4). For both genders, sexual intercourse is more frequent among black youth, followed in descending order by Hispanic youth and white youth (2–5). In general, males become sexually active at younger ages than do females.

Unfortunately, a substantial amount of adolescent sexual behavior appears to be unwanted and is the result of sexual assault. For example, in a large study of students attending secondary schools in Los Angeles, 18% of females and 12% of males reported that they had engaged in an unwanted sexual encounter (6). The sexual encounter had first occurred prior to age 12 for 39% of adolescents, and for over half of the group, it began between the ages of 13 and 16. Date rape comprised 31% of unwanted sexual encounters. Other epidemiological studies support the figure that approximately 15% of college women and 12% of high school adolescents have experienced unwanted sexual encounters (7–9). These studies usually fail to distinguish assault by family members (i.e., incest) from sexual assault by non-family members. Since the greatest occurrence of nonvoluntary sexual behavior is during middle to late adolescence, however, the rates reported above probably represent sexual assault rather than incest.

Moore and associates, in an analysis of data from a national survey, found that among 20-year-old youths approximately 13% of white females, 8% of black females, 2% of white males, and 6% of black males reported they had been raped or had been forced to engage in sexual intercourse (9). Factors associated with the likelihood of experiencing nonvoluntary intercourse among white females were separation from parents before age 16; physical, emotional, or mental limitation during childhood; and parental history of heavy drinking, drug use, or smoking. Data were not analyzed for black females or for males.

To promote responsible sexual behavior, it is especially important to reach adolescents—especially young adolescents—prior to their involvement in sexual intercourse. Adolescents who initiate sexual intercourse at younger ages are more likely to have a greater frequency of intercourse and a greater number of sexual partners (5, 10, 11). Young sexually active adolescents are also substantially less likely than older adolescents to initiate contraception. Approximately 40% of 15-year-old females wait more than 12 months after first intercourse to start contraception, while 35% of females age 15–17 and 15% of those age 18–19 postpone contraception more than one year (2, 11). Also, 60% of female adolescents under age 15 who become sexually active do not use contraception at first intercourse, compared with approximately 50% of adolescents who become sexually active at older ages.

The need for early intervention with all adolescents, but especially young adolescents, is further emphasized by data investigating the interval between initiation of first intercourse and pregnancy. Zabin and associates analyzed data from a national sample of adolescents who had a premarital pregnancy (12). Twenty-four percent of adolescents who were less than age 15 at first intercourse had become pregnant within 12 months of becoming sexually active (22% of white adolescents and 36% of black adolescents). Comparable figures for older adolescents were 24% (26% white and 30% black) for adolescents who had first intercourse at age 16–17; and 17% (18% white and 17% black) for adolescents age 18–19.

Contraceptive use by adolescents at first and subsequent intercourse has increased substantially over the past decade, primarily because of increased use of condoms (11, 13, 14). Overall, 78% of females and males have used a method of contraception at last intercourse (4). This rate is greatest for white adolescents, followed by black and Hispanic youth. Among those who use contraception, birth control pills are used by over 60% percent of sexually active, never-married females between 15 and 19 years old (15). Over 20% of this group report using condoms. The use of condoms is especially important because of the protection provided against STDs, including HIV infection.

Although the trend toward more frequent use of condoms is encouraging, adolescents most at risk for unintended pregnancy and STDs—such as those who are younger, who have multiple sexual partners, or who have a history of prior noncompliance with a family planning method—are less consistent users of condoms than other adolescents (13, 14, 16–18). Data from a 1988 national survey suggest that 30% of adolescent males use condoms on a regular basis, almost 50% use them sometimes, and 20% report never using condoms (18). A large study of college students found that 25% of men and 16% of women always used a condom during sexual intercourse (19). Using data from a 1990 survey of high school students, the CDC found that 40% of females and 49% of males had used a condom at last sexual intercourse (20). Hispanic adolescents (both female and male) reported less use than did black or white adolescents. Use was greater among younger adolescents and among adolescents who reported having fewer sexual partners.

UNINTENDED PREGNANCY

Over one million adolescents conceive each year. Of these, approximately 13% will have a miscarriage, 40% an elective abortion, and 47% a live birth (21). Although the distribution of pregnancy outcomes are similar for racial and ethnic groups, adolescents younger than 18 are substantially more likely to terminate their pregnancy with an induced abortion than are adolescents 18 and older. Overall, adolescents now account for 27% of all elective abortions performed in the United States (21).

Pregnancy rates for adolescents—defined as the rate of live births plus the rate of induced abortions per 1,000 females 15–19 years old—declined from the early 1970s to the mid-1980s and then began to rise slightly (21, 22). Despite the earlier decline, the United States still has the highest adolescent pregnancy rate and the highest birth rate of any Western nation (23). Nonwhite adolescents have double the pregnancy rate of white adolescents (21). During the early 1980s, the birth rate for females age 15–19 declined from 53 per 1,000 in 1980 to 50.6 per 1,000 in 1986 (24). Since 1986, however, births to adolescents have increased, and the 1989 birth rate of 58.1 per 1,000 is the highest recorded rate since the early 1970s. This increase has been especially large among adolescents younger than 18. Although the birth rate among adolescents under age 15 is low, adolescent mothers under 15—a group at especially high risk of adverse medical and psychosocial consequences—had 11,486 births in 1989.

The trend over the past several decades has been toward adolescents not marrying prior to delivery. In 1970, 30% of all births to adolescents occurred outside of marriage; this figure has now risen to 67% (24). Although the trend occurred for all adolescents, it was especially striking for black adolescents. In 1989, 92% of births to black adolescent mothers occurred outside of marriage. Single adolescent parenthood has significant impact on the ability of young mothers to financially support their families, complete school and, in general, maintain social relationships (25).

Although the rates of sexual intercourse have risen dramatically over the past two decades, the rates of pregnancies among adolescents at risk for pregnancy (i.e., those who are sexually active) have actually declined. This relationship is shown in Figure 7.1.

The conclusion drawn from Figure 7.1 is that, although adolescent pregnancy rates are high, preventive interventions must be having some positive effect, because the increase in the pregnancy rate has not kept pace with the increased rate of sexual activity.

Not surprisingly, the individual and societal costs of unintended adolescent pregnancy are large. The Center for Population Options in 1989 estimated societal costs of adolescent parenthood at $21.55 billion (26). Approximately 50% of these costs are for Aid to Families with Dependent Children (AFDC), 35% are for food stamps, and 15% are for Medicaid. Pregnant adolescents are more likely than other mothers to deliver low-birth-weight infants (27). This appears to be more related to social and environmental factors, such as poor nutrition and late prenatal care, than to physiological immaturity (28). Rapid repeat pregnancy also adversely affects obstetrical outcome of adolescents (28). Approximately 25% of adolescents age 16 and younger, and 20% of adolescents 17–18 have a second child within two years of having their first child (29). In addition to the effect on young mothers, early childbearing also has adverse effects on a young father's educational and vocational attainment, social and peer interactions, and marital relationship (30–32). Many adolescent parents do eventually succeed academically, vocationally, and socially, but they need strong support from parents, friends, and other community resources.

STDs, Including HIV Infection

Adolescents account for an estimated 3–6 million cases of sexually transmissible diseases each year (24, 33). Because GAPS addresses preventive ser-

Figure 7.1. Comparison of Trends in Sexual Intercourse and Pregnancy: Sexually Active Females

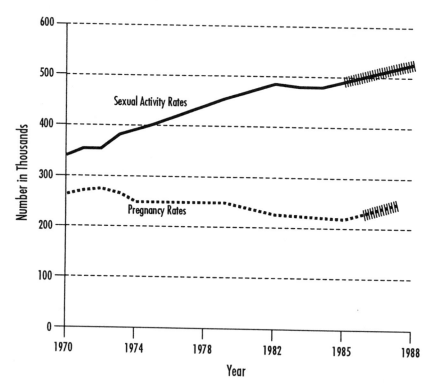

Source: U.S. Congress, Office of Technology Assessment, Adolescent Health—Vol. II: Background and the Effectiveness of Selected Prevention and Treatment Services. Washington, D.C., 1991:328.

vices directed at asymptomatic individuals, the discussion of STDs will focus on infections that cause significant morbidity and may be present, but without signs or symptoms. These infections include chlamydia, gonorrhea, syphilis, human papilloma virus, and HIV infection. Infection with hepatitis B virus (HBV) is discussed in Chapter 15.

The prevalence rates of chlamydia and gonorrhea among sexually active adolescents vary widely, with figures ranging from 9–35% for the former and 3–20% for the latter (34–40). The combination of large numbers of infected adolescents and the severe morbidity makes chlamydia and gonorrhea two of the major morbidities affecting adolescents. Chlamydia and gonorrhea cause a range of acute female genitourinary infections, including cervicitis, pelvic inflammatory disease, tubo-ovarian abscess, and infertility

(33). Among males, chlamydia and gonorrhea cause urethritis, proctitis, and epididymitis. However, most males, and many females, infected with either chlamydia or gonorrhea are asymptomatic (35, 36, 41). Systemic infections by either organism can lead to disseminated disease affecting joints, heart, and other organ systems (33). Treatments for chlamydia, gonorrhea, and syphilis are effective and have been described by the Centers for Disease Control and Prevention (42).

The rate of syphilis, which has increased among all age groups, doubled between 1975 and 1987 among adolescents (43). In 1980, 13% of the 27,204 cases of syphilis in the United States occurred among adolescents age 15–19, and 28% of cases were found among young adults age 20–24. The incubation period for syphilis varies from 9–90 days. Most adolescents, however, appear to present during the secondary stage of the infection, which occurs within six months of exposure (44). The history of a classic chancre lesion is often not reported by adolescents. Symptoms of secondary syphilis typically include lymphadenopathy and a rash that is truncal or located on the palms and soles. Syphilis in the secondary and tertiary phases of the disease can affect multiple organ systems and lead to serious medical disease. Since adolescents are often unaware they have syphilis, and since treponema pallidum is transmitted across the placenta, a major problem with this STD is the risk for congenital infection. Infants infected with syphilis incur a range of medical problems, from stillbirth to neurological impairment.

Condyloma acuminata, or genital warts, is a sexually transmissible disease caused by human papilloma virus (HPV). Study results document the large rise over the past decade in genital condyloma infections (45, 46). Although condyloma is not a reportable disease and is often asymptomatic, results of clinical and epidemiological studies suggest that HPV infection may be the most common viral STD among adolescents. Investigators have found 5–38% of sexually active adolescents had cytological evidence of HPV infection (47–49). Up to half of adults with genital condylomata have a coexisting infection with cervical papilloma virus (50).

Martinez and associates studied the relationships among clinical condyloma, abnormal cytological findings, and the recovery of human papillomavirus DNA in a group of 89 sexually active adolescents (51). Twelve adolescents had condyloma acuminata, while 24% had abnormal cytology from Pap smear and 13% had positive DNA from cervical scrapings. Among the adolescents with normal Pap smears, only 9% had vulvar warts and only 3% had DNA for HPV. Conversely, of adolescents with abnormal cytologies, 29% had genital warts and 48% had DNA for HPV. Adolescents may be especially susceptible to HPV because the columnar epithelium of the ectocervix that characterizes early puberty is more vulnerable to infection than the squamous epithelium that characterizes the cervical lining of adults (47). Condyloma transmission rate between sexual partners appears quite high (46, 52). In one study, over 40% of males who had sexual partners with genital warts had either genital condyloma acuminata or lesions showing histopathology consistent with HPV infection (53).

The major concern regarding HPV infection is the clinical and epidemiological evidence linking HPV cervical infection and lower genital track neoplasia (46, 52). The association between HPV and neoplastic changes is stronger for some HPV DNA types, such as 16 and 18, than for other DNA types. This is important because studies that control for sexual activity show an inconsistent relationship between a history of genital warts, which are usually caused by DNA types 6 and 11, and cervical neoplasia (46). A much stronger association is found when studies relate DNA types 16 and 18 to neoplasia.

Although HIV infections and AIDS are relatively rare among adolescents, the rates for these diseases are increasing rapidly. Studies of military recruits and job corp trainees found HIV infection in .33–.40 per 1,000 adolescents (54, 55). Seroprevalence is greater among males and minority groups. In a survey of adolescents attending 84 STD clinics, the median prevalence rate of HIV infection among heterosexual adolescents was 0.4% (56). Adolescent risk for HIV infection is predominantly due to unsafe sexual practices, rather than use of contaminated needles (57–59). Although the number of adolescents with AIDS is small, 20% of AIDS patients are in their mid-twenties and probably contracted the virus during their adolescence (55).

The magnitude of unmarried adolescents who are engaged in sexual behaviors that place them at risk for HIV infection has been recently studied by Seidman and associates (60). The dependent measure, risk for HIV infection, was having sexual intercourse with two or more partners in the previous three months. Using data from the National Survey of Family Growth, Seidman and associates found that 8.2% of females between age 15 and 19 were at risk for HIV infection, compared to 5.4% of females age 20–24 and 3.4% of those 25–29. White adolescents and adolescents who had their first sexual intercourse at less than 18 years were significantly more likely to have had multiple recent sexual partners than were black adolescents and adolescents who had their first sexual intercourse at age 18 or older.

Cervical Intraepithelial Neoplasia

In addition to the risks of unintended pregnancy and STD infections, adolescent females who engage in sexual intercourse are also at risk for developing cervical intraepithelial neoplasia (CIN). Studies conducted over the past several decades suggest that 2–3% of female adolescents age 15–19 have CIN (61–64). In a study of 194,069 adolescents age 15–19, Sadeghi and associates found that 1.94%, or 18.8 per 1,000 females, had CIN (61). Cervical biopsies were performed on 424 adolescents who had abnormal cytology. Of these adolescents 43%, or 10.7 per 1,000, had dysplasia and 14%, or 2.6 per 1,000, had carcinoma in situ.

There appears to be general agreement that the two major behavioral risk factors for abnormal cytology are young age at first sexual intercourse and multiple sexual partners (51, 65–68).

The other risk factor most consistently reported in the literature is infection with a sexually transmitted disease, especially HPV (66–68).

Co-morbidity

A recent major research finding is the association between sexual behavior and other health-risk behaviors. For example, in a study of over 1,500 junior high school students, Orr and associates found that sexually active adolescents, compared to those who were not sexually active, were 6.3 times more likely to have used alcohol, 4 times more likely to have used drugs other than marijuana, and 9.7 times more likely to have ridden with a driver who was using drugs (69). These ratios did not differ greatly by gender. Among 15-year-old youths in this study, 63% of males and 50% of females were both sexually active and using drugs.

Other investigators have also found moderately strong associations among sexual behavior, alcohol and drug use, smoking, delinquency, and poor school performance in adolescents of all ages (70–73). The relationships among alcohol use, sexual intercourse, and contraceptive use may be especially problematic; adolescent females who drink are less likely to use contraception at the time of first intercourse than are females who do not drink (74). In addition, adolescents who are heavy drinkers use condoms less frequently than do adolescents who are light drinkers or nondrinkers (14). Reasons for these associations among health-risk behaviors include: (1) adolescents who engage in various health-risk behaviors may have common psychological characteristics; (2) involvement in alcohol and drugs may reduce sexual inhibition; (3) sexual favors may be used to obtain drugs or money; and (4) adolescents who engage in these behaviors may be more emotionally troubled and seek out more deviant peer groups. Regardless of the reasons it is clear that some, but not all, adolescents engage in multiple behaviors that threaten their health. Preventive interventions directed at adolescents must, therefore, take into account these interactions.

JUSTIFICATION

How Can Physicians Best Promote Responsible Sexual Behavior, Including Abstinence?

There is a growing body of scientific information supporting the strategy that reducing risk for unintended pregnancy and STDs, including HIV infection, can be influenced by addressing: (1) how adolescents perceive their susceptibility to consequences if they fail to adopt desired behavior (e.g., don't use contraception) and how they perceive the benefits of desired behavior (e.g., prevention of pregnancy and STDs); (2) how strongly they feel that they can actually implement the desired behavior; and (3) their perception of how the desired behavior is viewed by peers, parents, and others (14, 16, 18, 75–77).

In contrast to other settings, where guidance is provided in groups or by written or audiovisual material, physicians can address each of these issues during a face-to-face office encounter. Because they are viewed by many adolescents as a highly authoritative source of information (78), physicians may be effective in using this trust to promote responsible sexual behavior. Support for this approach is provided by data from a statewide study conducted by Hingson and associates. From a random sample of almost 1,800 adolescents, the investigators found that students who had discussed AIDS with a physician were 1.7 times more likely than other adolescents to always use a condom (14). Because of opportunities provided in a clinical setting, several health advocates have called upon physicians to use office visits as an opportunity to promote responsible sexual behavior (14, 75).

Although increased knowledge may affect feelings of self-efficacy and how the adolescent perceives the benefits and costs of the desired behavior, it does not appear to have a strong direct effect on promoting responsible behavior (75, 77, 79–81). Physicians must also provide guidance to increase motivation and help adolescents develop the skills needed to make informed decisions. Some people express concern that discussing sexuality will lead adolescents to experimentation. Study results to date, however, fail to substantiate an association between sex education and an increase in sexual intercourse (81).

Physicians may increase contraception use by tailoring family planning services to meet the special needs of adolescents. For example, using an experimental design, Winter and associates demonstrated that female adolescents who received a special family planning protocol continued using the prescribed method of contraception more frequently and experienced fewer pregnancies at one year than did a control group of adolescents who received regular services from family planning clinics (82). This protocol included one-to-one education, visual aids, frequent and extended appointments, and involvement of the male partner in the family planning process.

In another study, Marcy and associates studied the effects of contraceptive counseling provided to a group of 122 unmarried, sexually active adolescent females age 13–18 (83). Subjects were randomly assigned to receive conventional counseling (involving assessment of contraceptive risk, discussion of methods of contraception, prescription of a method, and instructions regarding use) or developmental counseling (including conventional counseling but also stressing the adolescent's maturity, responsibility, and ability to make her own decisions regarding contraception). One year after the intervention, adolescents who received developmental counseling were substantially more effective users of contraception than were adolescents who received traditional counseling.

No studies to date have investigated whether health guidance provided in clinical settings is effective in reducing unsafe sexual behaviors. However, success with promoting safer sexual behavior, including abstinence, through a health education curriculum has been demonstrated by Kirby and associates (84). The school curriculum included teaching explicit norms against unprotected sexual intercourse, which could be accomplished by maintaining abstinence or by using contraception. Students who participated in the curriculum demonstrated increased knowledge about sexual issues and greater amounts of parent-child communication about abstinence and contraception when compared to a control group of students. Kirby and associates also found that youths in the study group who were abstinent at the time of the intervention, and subsequently engaged in sexual intercourse, were more likely to use contraception at the time of the 18-month follow-up than were adolescents in the control group, who were also abstinent initially. These findings were quite strong and did not differ by race or gender. Although no direct relation was found between parent-adolescent communication and unprotected intercourse, other researchers have found that parents, especially mothers, play a key role in promoting delayed sexual involvement of their daughters (85, 86). By providing parents with health guidance on the importance of discussing sexual issues with their adolescents, and how this can best be done (see Chapter 2), physicians may indirectly effect adolescent sexual behavior.

Results of a recent national study of over 8,000 parents with children between the ages of 10 and 17 suggest that physicians can impact parents' communication with adolescents about sexual issues (87). Seventy-six percent of parents who had read an AIDS-related brochure had talked with their adolescent about AIDS, compared to 57% of parents who had not read material on AIDS. Thirty-seven percent of parents who had received a brochure on AIDS obtained it from a health care provider.

What are the Most Effective Ways to Routinely Screen for STDs?

Urethral (males) and cervical (females) cultures are the most reliable ways to identify chlamydia and gonorrhea. However, diagnostic models using selected behavioral and clinical criteria can increase the cost-effectiveness of screening for chlamydia and gonorrhea among asymptomatic adolescents (34, 88–90). The length of time required to culture chlamydia and the relatively high cost of culture have led to the development of rapid immunological tests, such as direct immunofluorescent and enzyme immunoassay methods. These tests are less expensive than cultures, and provide quick and reliable results (39, 91, 92). Rapid assay measures appear to be a cost-effective screen for adolescent females who are at high risk for having a chlamydia infection. For example, Phillips estimated that using a rapid test as a routine screen for chlamydia would reduce future medical costs of the disease if local prevalence of infection was 7% or less, while screening with culture would reduce costs only if the frequency of the infection was greater than 14% (93). Trachtenberg estimated that using an antibody test to routinely screen asymptomatic females for chlamydia and treat those with a positive result would save $6 million in the first year alone if the prevalence of infection among females was greater than 2% (94).

Microscopic detection of pyuria has been used to identify males with urethritis who may have gonorrhea or chlamydia (95). Although effective as a screening measure, this procedure is relatively time-consuming and requires laboratory equipment. Urine leukocyte esterase (LE) screening, however, requires only a dipstick procedure and can be done quickly and inexpensively. Results of various studies indicate that urine leukocyte esterase has a sensitivity and specificity of approximately 80–90% for detecting pyuria among asymptomatic males (96–100). When compared with other tests for the detection of chlamydia, the LE test has a lower average cost-per-cure rate ($51) than does screening with culture ($414) or with direct smear fluorescent antibody ($192) (101).

Because of low rates of gonorrhea infection of the oral pharynx, only adolescents who give a history of having oral sex should be screened by pharyngeal culture for gonorrhea (102, 103). Similarly, because of relatively low rates of syphilis among the general adolescent population, screening tests for syphilis are usually only performed on special groups most at risk for infection. This includes adolescents who have had multiple or recurrent STDs, have had sex with more than one partner during the past six months, have exchanged sex for money or drugs, have had a sexual partner with a STD, or are males who have engaged in sex with other males (104). Sexually active adolescents who live in an area with a high rate of syphilis should also be tested.

Condylomata acuminata can usually be identified visually. If necessary, the presence of small genital lesions can be confirmed with acetic acid soaking (105). After several minutes soaking with a 3–5% acetic acid solution, condyloma appear as small white plaques. This whitening effect is also seen on epithelial surfaces that are healing or abraded. Cervical HPV infection is most often first suspected by cytological changes noted on a routine Pap smear. Colposcopy evaluation with biopsy is necessary to obtain a histological diagnosis and DNA type. Because of the large number of adolescents with genital HPV infections, only those females who have cervical condyloma or cytological dysplasia on Pap smear should receive colposcopy. Adolescents with genital condyloma acuminata should be treated and followed closely with repeat Pap smears.

HIV testing must be managed carefully because of the broad social and health implications of a positive test. CDC recommends that the ELISA test be used to screen for HIV infection, with presumptive positive results confirmed by follow-up tests (106). Because of the highly sensitive nature of the disease, GAPS recommends that HIV testing be done confidentially, following consent of the adolescent, and in conjunction with both pretest and posttest counseling (107).

CLINICAL APPLICATION

What constitutes responsible sexual behavior relates to various factors, including the age and developmental status of the adolescent, parental attitudes, cultural beliefs, and the nature of the behavior itself. For many adolescents, especially those who are younger and less mature physically and emotionally, responsible sexual behavior should consist of abstinence. "Second virginity," regardless of how short or how long this period might last, could be a goal that some adolescents elect. For older adolescents more capable of making decisions based on consideration of the potential effects of their behavior, a goal of responsible sexual behavior might be to prevent unintended pregnancy and STDs, including HIV infection. Having sexual relationships with multiple partners, selling sex for drugs or money, failing to use condoms and other contraceptive methods to prevent STDs and unintended pregnancy, and sexual exploitation are inappropriate behaviors regardless of age or developmental status.

Despite the circumstances surrounding sexual involvement, however, adolescents who choose to remain sexually active should be provided condoms and an appropriate method of contraception. Having condoms available in a medical setting may promote utilization by linking access to condoms with increase motivation and improved attitudes toward their use. The recurrence of STD among adolescents is high, especially within the first several months of the initial infection (108). Providing condoms to adolescents with a STD infection will help reduce the transmission to or reinfection from a sexual partner. Because of the association between health-compromising sexual behavior, poor self-esteem, and other health-risk behaviors, practitioners should be especially vigilant when discovering adolescents, especially young adolescents, who are sexually involved.

REFERENCES

1. Moore KA, Peterson JL, Furstenberg FF. Starting early: the antecedents of early, premarital intercourse. Paper presented at the 1984 annual meeting of the Population Association of American, Minneapolis, 1984.

2. Hofferth SL, Hayes CD. Risking the Future: Adolescent Sexuality, Pregnancy, and Childbearing (Vol. 2). Washington, DC: National Research Council, 1987.

3. US Congress, Office of Technology Assessment. Adolescent Health-Volume II: Background and the Effectiveness of Selected Prevention and Treatment Services. OTA-H-466. Washington, DC: US Government Printing Office, 1991:323–427.

4. Centers for Disease Control. Sexual behavior among high school students: United States, 1990. MMWR 1991;40:885–888.

5. Zelnik M, Shah F. First intercourse among young Americans. Fam Plann Perspect 1983;15:64–70.

6. Erickson PI, Rapkin AJ. Unwanted sexual experiences among middle and high school youth. J Adolesc Health 1991;12:319–325.

7. O'Keefe NK, Brockopp K, Chew E. Teen dating violence. Soc Work 1986;31:465–468.

8. Koss MP, Gidycz CA, Wisniewski N. The scope of rape: incidence and prevalence of sexual aggression and victimization in a national sample of higher education students. J Consult Clin Psychol 1987;55:162–170.

9. Moore KA, Nord CW, Peterson JL. Nonvoluntary sexual activity among adolescents. Fam Plann Perspect 1989;21:110–114.

10. Koyle PF, Jensen LC, Olsen J, Cundick B. Comparison of sexual behaviors among adolescents having an early, middle, and late first intercourse experience. Youth Soc 1989;20:461–476.

11. Mosher WD, McNally JW. Contraceptive use at first premarital intercourse: United States, 1965–1988. Fam Plann Perspect 1991;23:108–116.

12. Zabin LS, Kantner JF, Zelnik M. The risk of adolescent pregnancy in the first months of intercourse. Fam Plann Perspect 1979;11:215–222.

13. Hingson R, Strunin L, Berlin B. Acquired immunodeficiency syndrome transmission: changes in knowledge and behaviors among teenagers, Massachusetts statewide surveys, 1986 to 1988. Pediatrics 1990;85:24–29.

14. Hingson RW, Strunin L, Berlin BM, Heeren T. Beliefs about AIDS, use of alcohol and drugs, and unprotected sex among Massachusetts adolescents. Am J Public Health 1990;80:295–299.

15. Bachrach CA. Contraceptive practice among American women, 1973–1982. Fam Plann Perspect 1984;16:253–259.

16. Orr DP, Langefeld CD, Katz BP, et al. Factors associated with condom use among sexually active female adolescents. J Pediatr 1992;120:311–317.

17. Sonenstein FL, Pleck JH, Ku LC. Sexual activity, condom use and AIDS awareness among adolescent males. Fam Plann Perspect 1989;21:152–158.

18. Pleck JH, Sonenstein FL, Ku LC. Adolescent males' condom use: relationships between perceived cost-benefits and consistency. J Marr Fam 1991;53:733–745.

19. MacDonald NE, Wells GA, Fisher WA, et al. High-risk STD/HIV behavior among college students. JAMA 1990;263:3155–3159.

20. Centers for Disease Control. Selected behaviors that increase risk for HIV infection among high school students: United States, 1990. MMWR 1992;41:231, 237–240.

21. Ventura SJ, Taffel SM, Mosher WD. Estimates of pregnancies and pregnancy rates for the United States, 1976–1985. Am J Public Health 1988;78:504–511.

22. Maciak BJ, Spitz AM, Strauss LT, Morris L, Warren CW, Marks JS. Pregnancy and birth rates among sexually experienced US teenagers: 1974, 1980, and 1983. JAMA 1987;258:2069–2071.

23. Jones EF, Forrest JD, Goldman N, et al. Teenage pregnancy in developed countries: determinants and policy implications. Fam Plann Perspect 1985;17:53–63.

24. Facts at A Glance. Washington, DC: Child Trends, 1992.

25. Furstenberg FF, Brooks-Gunn J, Morgan SP. Adolescent mothers and their children in later life. Fam Plann Perspect 1987;19:142–151.

26. Armstrong E, Waszak C. Teenage Pregnancy and Too-Early Childbearing: Public Costs, Personal Consequences. Washington, DC: The Center for Population Options, 1990.

27. Lee K, Ferguson RM, Corpuz M, Gartner LM. Maternal age and incidence of low birth weight at term: a population study. Am J Obstet Gynecol 1988;158:84–89.

28. Elster A. The effect of maternal age, parity, and prenatal care on perinatal outcome of adolescent mothers. Am J Obstet Gynecol 1984;199:845–847.

29. Mott FL. The pace of repeated childbearing among young American mothers. Fam Plann Perspect 1986;18:5–12.

30. Hardy JB, Duggan AK. Teenage fathers and the fathers of infants of urban, teenage mothers. Am J Public Health 1988;78:919–922.

31. Teti DM, Lamb ME, Elster AB. Long-range socioeconomic and marital consequences of adolescent marriage in three cohorts of adult males. J Marr Fam 1987;49:499–506.

32. Marsiglio W. Teenage fatherhood: high school completion and education attainment. In: Elster AB, Lamb ME, eds. Adolescent Fatherhood. Hillsdale, NJ: Lawrence Erlbaum, 1986:67–87.

33. Shafer MA. Sexually transmitted disease syndromes. In: McAnarney ER, Kreipe R, Orr D, Comerci G, eds. Textbook of Adolescent Medicine. Philadelphia: WB Saunders Co, 1992:696–710.

34. Addiss DG, Vaughn ML, Holzhueter MA, Bakken LL, Davis JP. Selective screening for chlamydia trichomatous infection in nonurban family planning clinics in Wisconsin. Fam Plann Perspect 1987;19:252–256.

35. Saltz GR, Linnemann CC, Brookman RR, Raugh JL. Chlamydia trachomatous cervical infections in female adolescents. J Pediatr 1981;98:981–985.

36. Golden N, Hammerschlag M, Neuhoff S, Gleyzer A. Prevalence of chlamydia trichomatous cervical infection in female adolescents. Am J Dis Child 1984;138:562–564.

37. Chacko MR, Lovchik JC. Chlamydia trichomatous infection in sexually active adolescents: prevalence and risk factors. Pediatrics 1984;73:836–840.

38. Soren K, Willis E. Chlamydia and the adolescent girl. The enzyme immunoassay as a screening tool. Am J Dis Child 1989;143:51–54.

39. Shafer MA, Vaughan E, Lipkin ES, Mosicki BA, Schachter J. Evaluation of fluorescein-conjugated monoclonal antibody test to detect chlamydia trichomatous endocervical infections in adolescent girls. J Pediatr 1986;108:779–783.

40. Johnson BA, Poses RM, Fortner CA, Meier FA, Dalton HP. Derivation and validation of a clinical diagnostic model for chlamydia cervical infection in university women. JAMA 1990;264:3161–3165.

41. Handsfield HH, Lipman TO, Harnisch JP, Tronca E, Holmes KK. Asymptomatic gonorrhea in men: diagnosis, natural course, prevalence, and significance. N Engl J Med 1974;290:117–123.

42. Centers for Disease Control. 1989 sexually transmitted disease treatment guidelines. MMWR 1989;38(No. S-8):1–43.

43. Shafer MA, Moscicki AB. Sexually transmitted diseases. In: Hendee WR, ed. The Health of Adolescents. San Francisco: Jossey Bass, 1991:211–249.

44. Silber TJ, Niland NF. The clinical spectrum of syphilis in adolescence. J Adolesc Health Care 1984;5:112–116.

45. Johnson RE, Nahmias AJ, Magder LS, Lee FK, Brooks CA, Snowden CB. A seroepidemiologic survey of the prevalence of herpes simplex virus type 2 infection in the United States. N Engl J Med 1989;321:7–12.

46. Koutsky LA, Galloway DA, Holmes KK. Epidemiology of genital human papilloma virus infection. Epidemiol Rev 1988;10:122–163.

47. Rosenfeld WD, Vermund SH, Wentz SJ, Burk RD. High prevalence rate of human papilloma virus infection and association with abnormal papanicolaou smears in sexually active adolescents. Am J Dis Child 1989;143:1443–1447.

48. Zaninetti P, Franceschi S, Baccolo M. Characteristics of women under 20 with cervical intraepithelial neoplasia. Int J Epidemiol 1986;15:477–482.

49. Fisher M, Rosenfeld WD, Burk RD. Cervicovaginal human papilloma virus infection in suburban adolescents and young adults. J Pediatr 1991;119:821–825.

50. Walker PG, Calley NV, Grugg C. Abnormalities of the uterine cervix in women with vulvar warts. Br J Vener Dis 1983;59:120–126.

51. Martinez J, Smith R, Farmer M, Resau J, Alger L, et al. High prevalence of genital tract papillomavirus infection in female adolescents. Pediatrics 1988;82:604–608.

52. Syrjanen K, Vayrynen M, Saariloski S, et al. Natural history of cervical human papilloma virus (HPV) infections based on prospective follow-up. Br J Obstet Gynecol 1985;92:1086–1092.

53. Barrasso R, De Brux J, Croissant O, Orth G. High prevalence of papilloma virus-associated penile intraepithelial neoplasia in sexual partners of women with cervical intraepithelial neoplasia. N Engl J Med 1987;317:916–923.

54. Burke DS, Brundage JF, Goldenbaum M, et al. Human immunodeficiency virus infections in teenagers: seroprevalence among applicants for US military service. JAMA 1990;263:2074–2077.

55. Centers for Disease Control. Human immunodeficiency virus infection in the United States: a review of current knowledge. MMWR 1987;36(No. S-6):1–48.

56. Wendell DA, Onorato IM, McCray E, Allen DM, Sweeney PA. Youth at risk: sex, drugs, and human immunodeficiency virus. Am J Dis Child 1992;146:76–81.

57. Goodman E, Cohall AT. Acquired immunodeficiency syndrome and adolescents: knowledge, attitudes, beliefs, and behaviors in a New York City adolescent minority population. Pediatrics 1989;84:36–42.

58. Vermund SH, Hein K, Gayle HD, Cary JM, Thomas PA, Drucker E. Acquired immunodeficiency syndrome among adolescents. Am J Dis Child 1989;143:1220–1225.

59. Stiffman AR, Earls F. Behavioral risks for human immunodeficiency virus infection in adolescent medicine patients. Pediatrics 1990;85:303–310.

60. Seidman SN, Mosher WD, Aral SO. Women with multiple sexual partners: United States, 1988. Am J Public Health 1992;82:1388–1394.

61. Sadeghi SB, Hsieh EW, Gunn SW. Prevalence of cervical intraepithelial neoplasia in sexually active teenagers and young adults. Am J Obstet Gynecol 1984;148:726–729.

62. Fields C, Restivo RM, Brown MC. Experience in mass Papanicolaou screening and cytologic observations of teenage girls. Am J Obstet Gynecol 1976;124:730–734.

63. Kaufman RH, Burmeister RE, Spjut HJ. Cervial cytology in the teenage patient. Am J Obstet Gynecol 1970;108:515–519

64. Schydlower M, Greenberg H, Patterson PH. Adolescents with abnormal cervial cytology. Clin Pediatr 1981;20:723–726.

65. Wright VC, Riopelle MA. Age at beginning of coitus versus chronologic age as a basis for Papanicolaou smear screening: an analysis of 747 cases of preinvasive disease. Am J Obstet Gynecol 1984;149:824–830.

66. Zaninetti P, Franceschi S, Baccolo M, Bonazzi B, Gottardi G, Serraino D. Characteristics of women under 20 with cervical intraepithelial neoplasia. Int J Epidemiol 1986;15:477-482.

67. Moscicki AB, Winkler B, Irwin CE, Schachter J. Differences in biologic maturation, sexual behavior, and sexually transmitted disease between adolescents with and without cervical intraepithelial neoplasia. J Pediatr 1989;115:487–493.

68. Roye CF. Abnormal cervial cytology in adolescents: a literature review. J Adolesc Health 1992;13:643–650.

69. Orr DP, Beiter M, Ingersoll G. Premature sexual activity as an indicator of psychosocial risk. Pediatrics 1991;87:141–147.

70. Yamaguchi K, Kandel D. Drug use and other determinants of premarital pregnancy and its outcome: a dynamic analysis of competing life events. J Marr Fam 1987;49:257–270.

71. Elster AB, Ketterlinus RD, Lamb ME. The association between parenthood and problem behavior in a national sample of adolescent women. Pediatrics 1990;85:1044–1050.

72. Elster AB, Lamb ME, Tavare J. Association between behavioral and school problems and fatherhood in a national sample of adolescent youths. J Pediatr 1987;111:932–936.

73. Donovan JE, Jessor R. Structure of problem behavior in adolescence and young adulthood. J Consult Clin Psychol 1985;53:890–904.

74. Flanigan BJ, Hitch MA. Alcohol use, sexual intercourse, and contraception: an exploratory study. J Alcoh Drug Ed 1986;31:6–40.

75. DiClemente RJ, Drubin M, Siegel D, Krasnovsky F, Lazarus N, Comacho T. Determinants of condom use among junior high school students in a minority, inner-city school district. Pediatrics 1992;89:197–202.

76. Engquist KB, Parcel GS. Attitudes, norms, and self-efficacy. A model of adolescents' HIV-related sexual risk behavior. Health Educ Q 1992;19:263–277.

77. Shafer MA, Boyer CB. Psychosocial and behavioral factors associated with risk of sexually transmitted diseases, including human immunodeficiency virus infection, among urban high school students. J Pediatr 1991;119:826–833.

78. Helgerson SD, Peterson LR, and the AIDS Education Study Group. Acquired immunodeficiency syndrome and secondary school students: their knowledge is limited and they want to learn more. Pediatrics 1988;81:350–355.

79. Weisman CS, Nathanson CA, Ensminger M, Teitelbaum MA, Robinson JC, Plichta S. AIDS knowledge, perceived risk and prevention among adolescent clients of a family planning clinic. Fam Plann Perspect 1989;21:213–217.

80. DuRant RH, Sanders JM, Jay S, Levinson R. Analysis of contraceptive behavior of sexually active female adolescents in the United States. J Pediatr 1988;113:930–936.

81. Dawson DA. The effects of sex education on adolescent behavior. Fam Plann Perspect 1986;18:162–170.

82. Winter L, Breckenmaker LC. Tailoring family planning services to the special needs of adolescents. Fam Plann Perspect 1991;23:24–30.

83. Marcy SA, Brown JS, Danielson R. Contraceptive use by adolescent females in relation to knowledge, and to time and method of contraceptive counseling. Res Nurs Health 1983;6:175–182.

84. Kirby D, Barth RP, Leland N, Fetro JV. Reducing the risk: impact of a new curriculum on sexual risk-taking. Fam Plann Perspect 1991;23:253–263.

85. Spanier GB. Sources of sex information and premarital sexual behavior. J Sex Res 1977;13:73–88.

86. Inazu JK, Fox GL. Maternal influence on the sexual behavior of teen-age daughters. J Fam Issues 1980;1:81–102.

87. Jason J, Colclough G, Gentry EM. The pediatrician's role in encouraging parent-child communication about the acquired immunodeficiency syndrome. Am J Dis Child 1992;146:869–875.

88. Remafedi G, Abdalian SE. Clinical predictors of chlamydia trichomatous endocervicitis in adolescent women. Am J Dis Child 1989;143:1437–1442.

89. Handsfield HH, Jasman LL, Roberts PL, Hanbson VW, Kothenbeitel RL, Stamm WE. Criteria for selective screening for chlamydia trichomatous infection in women attending family planning clinics. JAMA 1986;255:1730–1734.

90. Nettleman MD, Jones RB, Roberts SD, et al. Cost-effectiveness of culturing for chlamydia trichomatous: a study in a clinic for sexually transmitted disease. Ann Intern Med 1986;105:189–196.

91. Stamm WE, Harrison HR, Alexander ER. Diagnosis of chlamydia trichomatous infections by direct immunofluorescence staining of genital secretions: a multicenter trial. Ann Intern Med 1984;101:638–641.

92. Neinstein LS, Rabinovitz S. Detection of chlamydia trichomatous: a study of the direct immunofluorescence technique and a review of the diagnostic limitations. J Adolesc Health Care 1988;10:10–15.

93. Phillips RS, Aronson MD, Taylor WC, Safran C. Should tests for chlamydia trichomatous cervical infection be done during routine gynecologic visits? Ann Intern Med 1987;107:188–194.

94. Trachtenberg AI, Washington AE, Halldorson S. A cost-based decision analysis for chlamydia screening in California family planning clinics. Obstet Gynecol 1988;71:101–108.

95. Adger H, Sweet RL, Shafer MA, Schachter J. Screening for chlamydia trichomatous and neisseria gonorrhea in adolescent males: value of first-catch urine examination. Lancet 1984Ct 27:944–945.

96. Shafer MA, Schacter J, Moscicki AB, et al. Urinary leukocyte esterase screening test for asymptomatic chlamydia and gonococcal infections in males. JAMA 1989;262:2562–2566.

97. Werner MJ, Biro F. Urinary leukocyte esterase screening for asymptomatic sexually transmitted disease in adolescent males. J Adolesc Health 1991;12:326–328.

98. Woods ER, Galvez LM, Talis AL, Emans SJ. First catch urine sediment for chlamydia trichomatous and neisseria gonorrhoea culture in adolescent males with pyuria. J Adolesc Health 1991;12:329–334.

99. O'Brien SF, Bell TA, Farrow JA. Use of a leukocyte esterase dipstick to detect chlamydia trichomatous and neisseria gonorrhea urethritis in asymptomatic adolescent male detainees. Am J Public Health 1988;78:1583–1584.

100. Sadof MD, Woods ER, Emans SJ. Dipstick leukocyte esterase activity in first-catch urine specimens. JAMA 1987;258:1932–1934.

101. Randolph AG, Washington AE. Screening for chlamydia trichomatous in adolescent males: a cost-based decision analysis. Am J Public Health 1990;80:545–550.

102. Brown RT, Lossick JG, Mosure DJ, Smeltzer MP, Cromer BA. Pharyngeal gonorrhea screening in adolescents: is it necessary? Pediatrics 1989;84:623–625.

103. Rooshvarg LB, Lovchik JC. Screening for pharyngeal gonorrhea in adolescents: a reexamination. J Adolesc Health 1991;12:269–272.

104. Shew ML, Fortenberry JD. Syphilis screening in adolescents. J Adolesc Health 1992;13:303–305.

105. American College of Obstetricians and Gynecologists. Genital human papillomavirus infections. ACOG Technology Bulletin 1987;105:1–4.

106. Centers for Disease Control. Guidelines for HIV Testing Services for Inpatients and Outpatients in Acute-Care Hospital Settings. Draft document, September, 1992.

107. Bresolin LB, Rinaldi RC. Human immunodeficiency virus blood test counseling for adolescents. Arch Fam Med 1993;2:673–676.

108. Blythe MJ, Katz BP, Batteiger BE, Ganser JA, Jones RB. Recurrent genitourinary chlamydial infections in sexually active female adolescents. J Pediatr 1992;121:487–493.

CHAPTER 8

Rationale and Recommendation: Hypertension

PREVENTION STRATEGY

In order to detect early hypertension, blood pressure should be taken on all adolescents annually. Because of the need to ensure accuracy and consistency in the diagnosis of hypertension, GAPS recommends physicians follow the clinical protocol developed by the Second Task Force on Blood Pressure Control in Children. This protocol distinguishes two levels of blood pressure: (1) true hypertension, which is systolic or diastolic blood pressure at or above the 95th percentile for age and sex and (2) "high normal" blood pressure, which is a level between the 90th and 95th percentile for age and sex. Baseline blood pressure should be based on measurements repeated at three different times within one month, under similar physical conditions. Adolescents with true hypertension should have a complete medical evaluation to establish treatment options. Adolescent obesity is related to elevated blood pressure levels. The physician guideline for counseling about healthy diet is addressed in GAPS Recommendation 7, while screening for obesity is addressed in Recommendation 13. Physician guidelines for screening for hypertension are included in GAPS Recommendation 11.

DISCUSSION

Blood pressure, especially systolic pressure, increases from the onset of adolescence and continues to rise until the end of pubertal growth (1–3). This trend appears related to increases in height, weight, and sexual maturation, and is noted more among males than females (3–6).

Approximately 1% of adolescents have sustained hypertension, defined as blood pressure greater than the 95th percentile of the standards set by the National Heart, Lung, and Blood Institute Second Task Force on Blood

Pressure Control in Children (2, 3, 7). This rate varies by gender, but not by race. Transient elevated blood pressure, also known as labile hypertension, may occur in up to 13% of adolescents (1, 2, 8). Although sustained hypertension among youth is relatively uncommon, the detection of hypertension during adolescence attracts a great deal of medical attention because hypertension is one of the major preventable factors contributing to the development of adult cardiovascular disease (9). In addition, even mild essential hypertension appears to have subtle cardiovascular effects during adolescence (10).

The National Heart, Lung, and Blood Institute has commissioned two reports on blood pressure in children. The first report was released in 1977; a revised report was released in 1987 (3). The objectives of the Report of the Second Task Force on Blood Pressure Control in Children—1987 were to: (1) determine the proper technique to measure blood pressure; (2) use existing data to prepare blood pressure distribution curves; (3) recommend blood pressure ranges representing normal, high normal, and hypertension; (4) present a scheme for detecting true hypertension; (5) identify diagnostic steps to evaluate someone with hypertension; and (6) identify effective non-pharmacological and pharmacological treatment strategies. Data for the report were taken from nine studies involving over 70,000 children of various ethnic groups and ages. The GAPS national scientific advisory board chose to use the recommendations developed by Second Task Force because of the scientific rigor with which they were developed.

JUSTIFICATION

The recommendation for screening for hypertension in adolescents is justified by conclusions derived from research data on the continuity between adolescent and adult hypertension, the ability to identify adolescent hypertension accurately, and the effectiveness of pharmacological and non-pharmacological treatment modalities for adolescent hypertension.

Does Hypertension Identified During Adolescence Track into Adulthood?

The rationale for early identification of adolescent hypertension is supported by data from various longitudinal studies demonstrating that blood pressure during childhood and adolescence remains at the same relative level over several decades (10–14). For example, in the Fels Longitudinal Growth Study, systolic blood pressure in male subjects at age 9 was significantly correlated with values 30 years later (14). Initial blood pressure at age 9 and the rate of change in blood pressure between age 9 and age 18, when taken together, accounted for approximately 20% of the variation in systolic blood pressure at age 30 (14). Data obtained serially from children enrolled in the Bogalusa Heart Study and in the Muscatine Study also suggest a moderately strong correlation between repeated measures of blood pressure over an 8–10-year period (11, 12). Even though individuals in these studies showed considerable variability in their blood pressure over time, there was a strong tendency for them to remain in similar quartiles compared to their peers. In the Muscatine Study, for example, 41% of children who were in the upper quartile for systolic blood pressure and 34% of those in the upper quartile for diastolic blood pressure remained in the same quartiles over a 10-year period (12). Similar results were found in the Bogalusa Heart Study (11). Family history of high blood pressure and obesity are both highly associated with the way blood pressure tracks into adulthood (11–13).

Can Hypertension During Adolescence Be Identified Accurately?

Blood pressure measurements can be obtained reliably and consistently if proper methods and instruments are used (3). Errors can occur when a blood pressure cuff is too small for the adolescent's arm and when values are compared with inappropriate age and gender norms. The values in Table 8.1 were developed by the Second Task Force on Blood Pressure Control in Children and should be used when assessing blood pressure in adolescents.

Vacillation of blood pressure during adolescence may produce false-positive results. For example, Sinaiko and associates assessed blood pressure levels of over 14,000 students who were 10–15 years old (7). Only 25–30% of students who had elevated blood pressure during their initial screening still had elevated blood pressure when re-evaluated at a later date. Other studies have substantiated the need to obtain three to four screening blood pressure levels before diagnosing sustained hypertension (1, 2, 8).

Can Hypertension During Adolescence Be Treated Effectively?

Effective nonpharmacological treatment for adolescent hypertension includes weight reduction (for those who are obese), physical exercise, and dietary modification (3). Weight reduction has been shown, among both adult and adolescent populations, to have a beneficial effect on lowering blood pressure (15–17). Using pooled data from five randomly controlled studies with obese adults, MacMahon and associates found that weight reduction had a modest but positive effect on lowering blood pressure among hypertensive patients (17). A weighted-mean difference in body weight of 9.2 kg resulted in a 3.1 mm/Hg drop in diastolic pressure and a 6.3 mm/Hg drop in systolic pressure. In another study, Rocchini and associates conducted a weight-loss intervention with 72 obese, normotensive adolescents

(18). Subjects were randomly assigned to one of three groups: diet and behavioral intervention; diet, behavioral, and exercise intervention; and no intervention. After 20 weeks, subjects in the two intervention groups had lost an average of 2.5 kg. During this interval, their systolic blood pressure declined by approximately 10 mm/Hg, while diastolic pressure declined by approximately 12 mm/Hg. Weight and blood pressure for the control group remained stable.

Dietary restriction of sodium is another nonpharmacological treatment approach that has been advocated by some health professionals as a way to lower blood pressure. According to the Second Task Force on Blood Pressure Control in Children, however, evidence supporting this intervention is not conclusive (3).

Results from epidemiological studies (19, 20) and from clinical trials (21) suggest that blood pressure levels of hypertensive adolescents can be reduced with increased levels of physical fitness. For example, Fraser and associates studied 228 students age 7–17 to determine the association between physical fitness and blood pressure (19). Even after adjusting for height, age, and body fat, adolescents' level of physical fitness was still significantly related to their level of systolic blood pressure. This association was found for both male and female adolescents. The authors hypothesize that increasing physical fitness may decrease systolic blood pressure by 4–5 mm/Hg in normal-weight youth. Hagberg and associates studied the effect of exercise training on reducing essential hypertension in 25 adolescents with an average age of 15.6 years (21). A group of 17 adolescents with essential hypertension who declined to participate in the training program were followed as a control group. Testing performed after six months of exercise training revealed that study subjects had an average reduction of 8 mm/Hg in systolic pressure and 5 mm/Hg in diastolic pressure. These changes occurred even though there was no change in body weight or body fat. When tested again nine months after cessation of exercise training, both systolic and diastolic pressures had returned to pretreatment levels. No change in blood pressure was noted for control group adolescents.

Antihypertensive medications are effective in adolescents with hypertension unresponsive to other treatments. These treatment modalities are reviewed in the Report of the Second Task Force on Blood Pressure Control in Children and, more recently, in the Report of the Joint National Committee on Detection, Evaluation, and Treatment of High Blood Pressure (3, 22).

Table 8.1. Blood Pressure Values (mm Hg) by Age and Gender

Age	Males (sitting)				Females (sitting)			
	Systolic		Diastolic		Systolic		Diastolic	
	90%	95%	90%	95%	90%	95%	90%	95%
11 yrs	119	123	76	80	119	123	77	81
12 yrs	122	126	77	81	122	126	78	82
13 yrs	124	128	77	81	124	128	78	83
14 yrs	126	130	78	82	125	129	81	85
15 yrs	129	133	79	83	126	130	82	86
16 yrs	132	136	81	85	127	131	81	85
17 yrs	133	138	83	87	127	132	81	84
18 yrs	136	140	84	88	127	132	80	84

Source: Second Task Force on Blood Pressure Control in Children. National Heart, Lung, and Blood Institute, 1987.

CLINICAL APPLICATION

The blood pressure values present in Table 8.1 should be used to determine whether an adolescent has hypertension, high normal blood pressure, or normal blood pressure. Adolescents with baseline blood pressure values above the 95th percentile for age and gender should be evaluated to determine if an obvious etiology can be found. For the majority of these adolescents no cause will be found and they can be assumed to have essential hypertension. Some, however, will have renal or cardiac disease.

Adolescents with blood pressure values between the 90th and 95th percentiles need to have multiple recordings (at least three) to determine their true baseline value. These recordings can be obtained by the school nurse, school-based health center, or by some facility convenient to the family. Adolescents with baseline values that remain in the high normal range should be counseled to lose weight (if obese) and increase their exercise. Care should be taken not to overdiagnose hypertension. Adolescents who have a blood pressure in the 90th to 95th percentile range, but who exceed the 90th percentile in height or lean body mass should be considered normotensive (3).

REFERENCES

1. Fixler DE, Laird WP. Validity of mass blood pressure screening in children. Pediatrics 1983;72:459–463.

2. Hediger ML, Schall JI, Katz SH, Gruskin AB, Eveleth PB. Resting blood pressure and pulse rate distributions in Black adolescents: the Philadelphia Blood Pressure Project. Pediatrics 1984;74:1016–1021.

3. National Heart, Lung, and Blood Institute. Report of the Second Task Force on Blood Pressure Control in Children—1987. Pediatrics 1987;79:1–25.

4. Londe S, Johanson A, Kronemer NS, Goldring D. Blood pressure and puberty. J Pediatr 1975;87:896–900.

5. Kozinetz CA. Sexual maturation and blood pressure levels of a biracial sample of girls. Am J Dis Child 1991;145:142–147.

6. Voors AW, Foster TA, Frerichs RR, Webber LS, Berenson GS. Studies of blood pressures in children, ages 5–14 years, in a total biracial community. Circulation 1976;54:319–327.

7. Sinaiko AR, Gomez-Marin O, Prineas RJ. Prevalence of "significant" hypertension in junior high school-aged children: the Children and Adolescent Blood Pressure Program. J Pediatr 1989;114:664–669.

8. Rames LK, Clarke WR, Conner WE. Normal blood pressures and the evolution of sustained blood pressure elevation in childhood: the Muscatine Study. Pediatrics 1978;61:245–251.

9. Kannel WB, Doyle JT, Ostfeld AML. The Framingham Study. Circulation 1984;70:157A–162A.

10. Sinaiko AR, Bass J, Gomez-Marin O, Prineas RJ. Cardiac status of adolescents tracking with high and low blood pressure since early childhood. J Hypertens 1987;4(suppl 5):378–380.

11. Shear CS, Burke GL, Freedman DS, Berenson GS. Value of childhood blood pressure measurements and family history in predicting future blood pressure status: results from 8 years of follow-up in the Bogalusa Heart Study. Pediatrics 1986;77:862–869.

12. Clarke WR, Woolson RF, Lauer RM. Changes in ponderosity and blood pressure in childhood: the Muscatine Study. Am J Epidemiol 1986;124:195–205.

13. Kotchen JM, Kotchen TA, Guthrie GP, Cottrill CM, McKean HE. Correlates of adolescent blood pressure at five-year follow-up. Hypertension 1980;2(suppl I):124–129.

14. Woynarowska B, Mukherjee D, Roche AF, Siervogel RM. Blood pressure changes during adolescence and subsequent adult blood pressure level. Hypertension 1985;7:695–701.

15. Brownwell KD, Kelman JH, Stunkard AJ. Treatment of obese children with and without their mothers: changes in weight and blood pressure. Pediatrics 1983;71:515–523.

16. Becque MD, Katch VL, Rocchini AP, Marks CR, Moorehead C. Coronary risk incidence of obese adolescents: reduction by exercise plus diet intervention. Pediatrics 1988;81:605–612.

17. MacMahon S, Cutler J, Brittain E, Higgins M. Obesity and hypertension: epidemiological and clinical issues. Eur Heart J 1987;8(suppl B):57–70.

18. Rocchini AP, Katch V, Anderson J, et al. Blood pressure in obese adolescents: effects of weight loss. Pediatrics 1988;82:16–23.

19. Fraser GE, Phillips RL, Harris R. Physical fitness and blood pressure in school children. Circulation 1983;67:405–411.

20. Fripp RR, Hodgson JL, Kwiterovich PO, Werner JC, Schuler HG, Whitman V. Aerobic capacity, obesity, and atherosclerotic risk factors in male adolescents. Pediatrics 1985;75:813–818.

21. Hagberg JM, Goldring D, Ehsani AA. Effect of exercise training on the blood pressure hemodynamic features of hypertensive adolescents. Am J Cardiol 1983;52:763–768.

22. Joint National Committee on Detection, Evaluation, and Treatment of High Blood Pressure. The fifth report of the Joint National Committee on Detection, Evaluation, and Treatment of High Blood Pressure (JNCU). Arch Intern Med 1993;153:154–183.

CHAPTER 9

Rationale and Recommendation: Hyperlipidemia

PREVENTION STRATEGY

GAPS recommends a selective testing procedure whereby adolescents at risk for hyperlipidemia are screened for serum cholesterol. This recommendation follows the protocol developed by the Expert Panel on Blood Cholesterol Levels in Children and Adolescents. Screening involves a three-step process: (1) assessment of family history for premature cardiovascular disease or hyperlipidemia, (2) screening for serum cholesterol level in adolescents with positive family history, and (3) analysis of serum lipids for adolescents with elevated cholesterol levels. Physicians may chose to screen adolescents for serum cholesterol when their family history is unknown or when they have other risk factors for premature cardiovascular disease (CVD), such as obesity, hypertension, and diabetes. Other risk factors for CVD include smoking and a diet high in cholesterol and fat.

The Expert Panel also recommends routine screening for serum cholesterol for any youth over 19 years who has not been previously tested. Unless serum cholesterol values are elevated, screening for hyperlipidemia only need be done once during adolescence. Physician guidelines for the other cardiovascular risk behaviors relating to diet, physical fitness, hypertension, obesity, and smoking are addressed, respectively, in GAPS Recommendations 7, 8, 11, 13, and 14. Guidelines for screening for hyperlipidemia are addressed in GAPS Recommendation 12.

DISCUSSION

Coronary artery disease (CAD) is the major cause of death among adults in the United States. Data from numerous studies and reports by expert panels lead to the conclusion that hypertension, hyperlipidemia, and smoking are each independent risk factors for the development of atherosclerosis, which is the pathophysiological process underlying CAD (1). Obesity and a sedentary lifestyle also are associated with CAD, but primarily through their negative effect on hypertension and hyperlipidemia (2–4).

An agenda for reducing premature adult morbidity and mortality is now focusing attention on cardiovascular risk reduction among children and adolescents (5). The rationale for this agenda is based on two concepts. First, although symptoms of atherosclerosis are rarely noted until adulthood, it appears that the pathogenic process begins much earlier in life (6, 7). Data from autopsy studies of adolescents and young adults demonstrate an association between the presence of aortic and coronary artery fibrous plaques and serum lipid levels (6, 7). Second, a substantial number of children and adolescents have risk factors that, presumably if reduced, would lower their risk of CAD later in life.

Results of several studies suggest that 23–35% of young adolescents have at least one risk factor for CAD (elevated serum cholesterol and triglyceride levels, hypertension, smoking, or obesity) and approximately 5–10% have two or more (8, 9). Behavior that begins during adolescence—such as smoking, eating foods high in fat and cholesterol, and leading a sedentary lifestyle—often persist throughout the life span unless interrupted by an intervention. Reducing an adolescent's later risk of premature cardiovascular disease necessitates early identification and control of hyperlipidemia and hypertension, as well as promotion of a healthy diet and lifestyle. The relatively high prevalence of hyperlipidemia within the adolescent population has brought attention to the need for general dietary counseling and serum cholesterol screening. In order to appropriately screen for hyperlipidemia, it is necessary to understand the normal developmental trajectory of serum cholesterol among adolescents.

Serum cholesterol rises slowly during childhood and peaks around the onset of accelerated linear growth (age 8–10 for girls and approximately age 10 for boys). Levels then decline during middle adolescence before rising again near the end of adolescence (10–13). This trend is greater for boys than for girls. In general, lipid levels are higher among black youth. Results from several studies indicate that approximately 20–30% of children and adolescents have a serum cholesterol level greater than 170 mg/dl, which is generally considered the upper limit of normal (10, 11, 13–15). Of these, approximately 10% have values above 200 mg/dl, and up to 0.5% have values greater than 230 mg/dl. Children in the latter group probably are heterozygous for familial hypercholesterolemia, a genetic disorder associated with greatly elevated levels of low-density lipoprotein (LDL) cholesterol and premature coronary artery disease.

The National Cholesterol Education Program (NCEP) was developed to help identify and coordinate a comprehensive national strategy that focuses on reducing premature deaths from cardiovascular disease. The Expert Panel on Blood Cholesterol Levels in Children and Adolescents was convened to develop a strategy, justified by a consensus of scientific information, that specifically targets risk reduction for the younger population. Their report, published in 1992, has been approved by the NCEP Coordinating Committee, which includes various national organizations and federal agencies (5).

The Expert Panel recommends two complementary approaches to reduce the risk of CVD: (1) a population approach to "lower the average level of blood cholesterol among all American children and adolescents through population-wide changes in nutrient intake and eating patterns" and (2) an individual approach of selective screening to "identify and treat children and adolescents who are at the greatest risk of having high blood cholesterol as adults and an increased risk of CHD [coronary heart disease]" (5). Because of the scientific basis upon which the recommendations were developed, and the public endorsement of the report by many national medical organizations, GAPS chose to support the recommendations of the Expert Panel.

JUSTIFICATION

Is It Possible to Identify, Through History and Selective Screening, Which Adolescents Are at Risk for Adult Coronary Artery Disease?

The results of numerous studies have demonstrated that lipoprotein levels of children mirror those of their parents (16–21). Moreover, adolescents with a parental history of cardiovascular disease are three to five times more likely to have abnormal lipid levels compared to other adolescents (16, 20, 21). This relationship appears to be stronger for white than black youths (16).

Although there is strong support for familial clustering of hyperlipidemia, using family history as the criteria for screening will miss a substantial number of adolescents with elevated serum lipid levels. Data from the Bogalusa Heart study were analyzed by Dennison and associates to determine the feasibility of using parental history of vascular disease (hypertension, heart attack, stroke, or diabetes) as a way to identify children with hyperlipidemia (16). This approach had modest success, with a sensitivity of 59% and a specificity of 67% for identifying white adolescents who had elevated lipids. Family history was somewhat less effective a predictor among black youths, with sensitivity and specificity values of 25% and 56%, respectively.

Steiner and associates, in a study of 1,000 adolescents, found that one-third to one-half of adolescents with elevated cholesterol, as detected by a universal screening program, would not have been screened using the recommendations for selective testing of serum cholesterol (22). Because of data such as these, some researchers advocate mass cholesterol screening for the entire population (13, 22). Still other researchers caution against any screening until adulthood because of the lack of solid evidence supporting the notion that lowering cholesterol during adolescence leads to the reduction of CAD. They also cite possible psychosocial risk from early diagnosis and treatment (23–25).

According to the Expert Panel, selective screening of children and adolescents who have parental cholesterol values of 240 mg/dl or higher will result in 25% of all youth being screened for hyperlipidemia (5). The Panel also estimated that 40.5% of adolescents with abnormally high LDL-cholesterol values (e.g., values equal to or greater than 130 mg/dl) would be identified with a selective screening approach. Although 59% of children and adolescents with elevated LDL cholesterol would be missed, the Panel concluded that their recommendations provide the best balance between the number of people screened and the number detected. The Panel also recognized, however, that the approach of using both population and selective screening strategies has not been demonstrated to be more effective than a universal screening strategy in the prevention of adult CHD (5).

Does a Person's Lipid Profile Remain Stable from Adolescence Through Adulthood?

Although values change substantially among many individuals, there is, nevertheless, a strong correlation between levels of serum cholesterol during adolescence and lipid values later in life. For example, in the Muscatine study of 1,391 children followed for over 10 years, Lauer and Clarke found that, of 70 children who had cholesterol levels greater than the 90th percentile, 71% had abnormal levels as adults (24). Conversely, of youths who had normal levels initially, only 17% had abnormal values as adults. Lauer and Clark calculated that 25–50% of the variance in adult levels of cholesterol was explained by the values during adolescence (26). In another longitudinal study, researchers found a high correlation between cholesterol levels obtained during early adolescence and levels obtained nine years (r 4 .52) and 16 years (r 4 .44) later (27, 28). Correlations were significantly greater for females than for males. Although the predictive value of cholesterol screening during childhood and early adolescence for identifying later hyperlipidemia is modest, some of the discrepancy between early and later values may be explained by changes in personal behaviors (i.e, smoking and exercise), diet, and oral contraceptive use (26, 28).

Can Hyperlipidemia Identified During Adolescence Be Modified?

Various treatments for hyperlipidemia include dietary modification, weight reduction, and lipid-lowering medications. Regular physical activity is also frequently suggested as a way to increase cardiovascular fitness and improve lipid profiles.

Treatment with dietary intervention appears to have a modest effect in improving lipid profiles among children and adolescents. Hanna and associates studied the effect of children and adolescents' problem-solving skills on adherence to a low-fat diet (29). Dietary counseling resulted in a 12% reduction of LDL cholesterol over a six-month period. The researchers also found adolescents' ability to generate coping strategies, a measure of problem-solving ability, predicted their current dietary habits. These results imply that, in addition to providing basic instruction, diet counseling should also help adolescents deal with social situations that affect adherence to a dietary regimen.

The beneficial effect of weight reduction on improving an adolescent's lipid profile has been shown in various studies (30, 31). This effect appears to be independent of change in level of fitness. For example, Epstein and associates found after six months of weight loss intervention, moderately strong correlations (r 4 .34–.53) between the amount of weight loss and the improvement in serum cholesterol, high-density lipoprotein (HDL) cholesterol, and triglycerides (30). Low correlations were noted between improvement in fitness and changes in serum lipid levels.

Studies of children treated with lipid-lowering drugs, with and without dietary alterations, have mainly been done in specialized lipid treatment centers. Although these approaches are effective in improving the lipid profile, they do not appear to produce optimal lipid levels. Long-term compliance has not been sufficiently studied (32–34).

In summary, dietary interventions and weight reduction appear to have moderate beneficial effects on improving the lipid profiles of adolescents with primary hyperlipidemia. Counseling to increase exercise might also be helpful (see Chapter 6). Care must be taken to ensure that dietary changes are appropriate to meet the nutritional needs of the growing adolescent.

Clinical Application

The primary management of adolescents with hyperlipidemia involves decreasing dietary saturated fatty acids, total fat, and cholesterol. The Expert Panel on Blood Cholesterol in Children and Adolescents provides preventive intervention recommendations based on an individual's lipid level (5). Because of the developmental changes in serum lipids and the different rates of pubertal growth among adolescents, care must be taken to individualize test results and interpret lipid values in association with each adolescent's stage of physical development. The following are the recommendations of the Expert Panel on how to manage adolescents with various lipid values:

Total cholesterol less than 170 mg/dl or LDL cholesterol less than 110 mg/dl:

Adolescents with these values should receive education on improving eating patterns (e.g., the same education advocated for the population-wide strategy), such as:

1. Eating a greater quantity of fruits, vegetables, grains;
2. Choosing low-fat dairy products, fish, poultry, and lean meat;
3. Eating "convenience foods" that are low in saturated fatty acids, total fat, and cholesterol.

Providers should also counsel patients to reduce other risk factors for CVD, such as smoking, physical inactivity, and obesity.

Total cholesterol from 170–199 mg/dl or LDL from 119–129 mg/dl:

Adolescents with these values require instruction on Step 1 Diet by either a physician, registered dietician, or other qualified health professional. This diet is designed to provide specific recommendations on reducing dietary intake of saturated fatty acids and cholesterol. The Step 1 Diet limits the intake of saturated fats to less than 10% of total calories, with no more than 30% of calories as fat and less than 300 mg of cholesterol per day. These adolescents should then be re-evaluated in one year. They should also be counseled to reduce other risk factors for CVD, such as refraining from smoking and increasing their exercise.

Total cholesterol greater than 199 mg/dl or LDL greater than 129 mg/dl:

Adolescents with these values are likely to have an inherited disorder of LDL metabolism and require more intensive clinical intervention. They should be instructed in Step 1 Diet, counseled to reduce other risk factors for CVD, and followed closely. If no improvement in lipid profile is seen after three months, they should be instructed in a Step 2 Diet. This diet limits the intake of saturated fats to less than 7% of total calories, with no more than 30% of calories as fat and the cholesterol amount reduced to less than 200 mg per day.

The Expert Panel recommends that drug therapy be considered if:

1. LDL cholesterol remains at 190 mg/dl or greater after dietary changes, or
2. LDL cholesterol remains at 160 mg/dl or greater and there is either (a) positive family history of premature CVD or (b) presence of two or more other CVD risk factors, even after attempts to reduce them.

REFERENCES

1. Consensus Conference of the National Institute of Heart, Lung, and Blood. Lowering blood cholesterol to prevent heart disease. JAMA 1985;253:2080–2086.
2. Khoury P, Morrison JA, Mellies MJ, Glueck CJ. Weight change since age 18 years on 30–55-year-old whites and blacks. JAMA 1983;250:3179–3187.
3. Van Itallie TB. Health implications of overweight and obesity in the United States. Ann Intern Med 1985;103:983–988.
4. Hubert HB, Feinleib M, McNamara PM, Castelli WP. Obesity as an independent risk factor for cardiovascular disease: a 26-year follow-up of participants in the Framingham Heart Study. Circulation 1983;67:968–977.
5. National Cholesterol Education Program. Report of the Expert Panel on Blood Cholesterol Levels in Children and Adolescents. Pediatrics 1992;89(suppl):525–584.
6. Newman WP III, Freedman DS, Voors AW. Relation of serum lipoprotein levels and systolic blood pressure to early atherosclerosis: the Bogalusa Heart Study. N Engl J Med 1986;314:138–144.
7. Newman WP III, Wattigney W, Berenson GS. Autopsy studies in US children and adolescents: relationship of risk factors to atherosclerotic lesions. Ann NY Acad Sci 1991;623:16–25.
8. Lauer RM, Connor WE, Leaverton PE, Eriter MA, Clarke WR. Coronary heart disease risk factors in school children. J Pediatr 1975;86:697–705.
9. Fripp RR, Hodgson JL, Kwiterovich PO, Werner JC, Schuler G, Whitman V. Aerobic capacity, obesity, and atherosclerotic risk factors in male adolescents. Pediatrics 1985;75:813–818.
10. Frerichs RR, Srinivasan SR, Webber LS, Berenson GS. Serum cholesterol and triglyceride levels in 3,446 children from a biracial community: the Bogalusa Heart Study. Circulation 1976;54:302–309.

11. Resnicow K, Morley-Kotchen J, Wynder E. Plasma cholesterol levels of 6,585 children in the United States: results of the Know Your Body screening in five states. Pediatrics 1989;84:969–976.

12. Cresanta JL, Srinivasan SR, Webber LS, Berenson GS. Serum lipid and lipoprotein cholesterol grids for cardiovascular risk screening of children. Am J Dis Child 1984;138:379–387.

13. Goff DC, Donker GA, Ragan JD, et al. Cholesterol screening in pediatric practice. Pediatrics 1991;88:250–258.

14. Srinivasan SR, Wattigney W, Webber LS, Berenson GS. Race and gender differences in serum lipoproteins of children, adolescents, and young adults—emergence of an adverse lipoprotein pattern in white males: the Bogalusa Heart Study. Prev Med 1991;20:671–684.

15. Glueck CJ, Mellies MJ, Tsang RC, Morrison JA. Risk factors for coronary artery disease in children: recognition, evaluation, and therapy. Pediatrics 1980;2:131–138.

16. Dennison BA, Kikuchi DA, Srinivasan SR, Webber LS, Berenson GS. Parental history of cardiovascular disease as an indication for screening for lipoprotein abnormalities in children. J Pediatr 1989;115:186–194.

17. Croft JB, Cresanta JL, Webber LS, et al. Cardiovascular risk in parents of children with extreme lipoprotein cholesterol levels: the Bogalusa Heart Study. South Med J 1988;81:341–349.

18. Lee J, Laurer RM, Clarke WR. Lipoproteins in the progeny of young men with coronary artery disease: children with increased risk. Pediatrics 1986;78:330–337.

19. Hennekens CH, Jese MJ, Klein BE, Gourley JE, Blumenthal S. Cholesterol among children of men with myocardial infarction. Pediatrics 1976;58:211–217.

20. Morrison JA, Kelly KA, Mellies ML, deGroot I, Glueck CJ. Parent-child associations at upper and lower ranges of plasma cholesterol and triglyceride levels. Pediatrics 1978;62:468–477.

21. Blumenthal S, Jesse MJ, Hennekens CH, Klein BE, Ferrer PL, Gourley JE. Risk factors for coronary artery disease in children of affected families. J Pediatr 1975;87:1187–1192.

22. Steiner NJ, Neinstein LS, Pennbridge J. Hypercholesterolemia in adolescents: effectiveness of screening strategies based on selected risk factors. Pediatrics 1991;88:269–275.

23. Newman TB, Browner WS, Hulley SB. The case against childhood cholesterol screening. JAMA 1990;264:3039–3043.

24. Lauer RM, Clarke WR. Use of cholesterol measurements in childhood for the prediction of adult hypercholesterolemia: the Muscatine Study. JAMA 1990;264:3034–3038.

25. Holtzman NA. The great god cholesterol (commentary). Pediatrics 1991;87:943–945.

26. Lauer RM, Lee J, Clarke WR. Factors affecting the relationship between childhood and adult cholesterol levels: the Muscatine Study. Pediatrics 1988;82:309–318.

27. Orchard TJ, Donahue RP, Kuller LH, Hodge PN, Drash AL. Cholesterol screening in children: does it predict adult hypercholesterolemia? The Beaver County experience. J Pediatr 1983;103:687–691.

28. Stuhldreher WL, Orchard TJ, Donahue RP, Kuller LH, Gloninger MF, Drash AL. Cholesterol screening in childhood: sixteen-year Beaver County Lipid Study experience. J Pediatr 1991;119:551–556.

29. Hanna KJ, Ewart CK, Kwiterovich PO. Child problem-solving competence, behavioral adjustment and adherence to lipid-lowering diet. Patient Ed Counsel 1990;16:119–131.

30. Epstein LH, Kuller LH, Wing RR, Valoski A, McCurely J. The effect of weight control on lipid changes in obese children. Am J Dis Child 1989;143:454–457.

31. Becque MD, Katch VL, Rocchini AP, Marks CR, Moorehead C. Coronary risk incidence of obese adolescents: reduction by exercise plus diet intervention. Pediatrics 1988;81:605–612.

32. Glucek CJ, Tsang RC, Fallat RW, Mellies M. Therapy of familial hypercholesterolemia in childhood: diet and cholestyramine resin for 24–36 months. Pediatrics 1977;59:433–441.

33. Stein EA. Treatment of familial hypercholesterolemia with drugs in children. Arteriosclerosis 1989;9(suppl I):145–151.

34. West RJ, Lloyd JK, Leonard JV. Long-term follow-up of children with familial hypercholesterolemia treated with cholestyramine. Lancet 1980; Oct 25:873–875.

CHAPTER 10

Rationale and Recommendations: Use of Tobacco Products

PREVENTION STRATEGY

GAPS recommends that all adolescents receive health education annually to promote avoidance of tobacco. Because of the rapid increase in use of tobacco products that occurs during adolescence, all youths should be asked annually about their use of cigarettes and smokeless tobacco. The interval between first use of tobacco and the development of nicotine addiction appears to be about two years. This time period offers an especially good "window of opportunity" for implementing a successful cessation program. Physician guidelines for health promotion regarding tobacco use are included in GAPS Recommendation 10. Guidelines for screening for tobacco use are included in Recommendation 14.

DISCUSSION

Great national attention is now directed at preventing smoking among adolescents because of the large numbers of youths who smoke, and because smoking habits usually begin early in life. Recent data from large national studies indicate that almost 16% of all adolescents smoke, and 22% of all adolescent males use smokeless tobacco (1, 2). These statistics are presented in Table 10.1.

As shown in Table 10.1, use of tobacco products varies by age and race. Adolescents who are older and who are white smoke and use smokeless tobacco at greater rates than do those who are younger and nonwhite. Rates of smoking do not vary, however, either by gender or by poverty status. By late adolescence, regular use of smokeless tobacco is approximately equal to regular smoking. Data from another study indicate that use of smokeless tobacco is especially prevalent among some groups of Native American adolescents (3).

Table 10.1. Cigarette and Smokeless Tobacco Use Among Adolescents, 1989

Group	Cigarette Use (%)				Smokeless Tobacco Use (%)	
	Never	Former	Casual	Regular	Never	Regular
Gender by Age						
Male						
12–13 years	73	0.5	24	3.5	87	12
14–15 years	54	2.0	31	13	72	19
16–18 years	37	2.5	34	26	55	25
Female						
12–13 years	78	0	18	4		
14–15 years	57	0.5	30	13		
16–18 years	41	2	33	24		
Race by Gender						
White						
Male	50	2	30	18	64	23
Female	53	1.5	28	17		
Black						
Male	61	0.5	31	7	88	7.5
Female	66	0	29	5		
Hispanic						
Male	57	1	30	12	87	9.5
Female	56	1.5	30	12		
Poverty Status						
In-Poverty	55	1.5	28	16		
Non-Poverty	53	1.5	29	16		

Source: 1. Moss AJ, Allen KF, Giovino GA, Mills SL. Recent trends in adolescent smoking, smoking-uptake
        correlates, and expectations about the future. Advance data from vital and health statistics;
        221. Hyattsville, MD: National Center for Health Statistics, 1992.
     2. Allen KF, Moss AJ, Giovino GA, Shopland DR, Pierce JP. Teenage tobacco use: data estimates from the
        Teenage Attitudes and Practices Survey, United States, 1989. Advance data from vital and health
        statistics; 224. Hyattsville, MD: National Center for Health Statistics, 1992.

The number of adolescent smokers fell from the mid-1970s until the early 1980s. Whereas nearly 30% of high school seniors were daily smokers in 1976, this figure declined to approximately 18% by 1984 and has remained stable since then (4). The decline in smoking was substantially smaller among adolescent females than among other age and gender groups. In fact, the percentage of female high school seniors who smoke is now equal to that of male high school seniors who smoke.

Although the overall number of adolescents who smoke has declined, smoking appears to start at younger ages than in previous generations (5). Initiation of tobacco use increases rapidly after age 11 and peaks between age 17–19 (6). The need for preventive intervention at young ages is underscored by the fact that, among high school seniors who smoke, 25% were smoking by the 6th grade and another 50% were smoking by the 8th grade (5).

Addiction to nicotine occurs gradually and some adolescents experiment with smoking and then stop (7, 8). This process appears to develop over a two-year period, and presents a window of opportunity during which preventive interventions may be especially effective. Once regular smoking patterns are established, however, they are hard to break. Smoking that begins during adolescence and young adulthood is strongly predictive ($r = .83$) of smoking during adulthood (9–11). Approximately 90% of all adult smokers began their habit prior to age 21, while 40–45% of adult females and 55–60% of adult males began smoking prior to age 18 (5). Adults with less than a high school education are substantially more likely to begin smoking during early adolescence than are those who have at least 12 years of formal education (6).

The long-term health consequences of cigarettes and passive smoking include coronary artery disease, lung cancer, and chronic obstructive pulmonary disease (5). Among adult females, smoking in conjunction with oral contraceptive use is associated with an increased risk for vascular problems and strokes (12). Smoking is responsible for 1-in-6 adult deaths in the United States and is the single most preventable cause of death (5). Approximately 35% of all cancer deaths among males and 18% of cancer deaths among females are attributable to smoking (13). Among adult smokers, lung cancer is the leading cause of death.

Precursors of adult cardiovascular disease caused by smoking are evident during adolescence. Youths who smoke have over 10% higher serum triglyceride and low-density lipoprotein (LDL) levels, and 8% lower high-density lipoprotein (HDL) levels than do nonsmoking adolescents (14, 15). In addition to effects on serum lipid profiles, smoking and exposure to passive smoke during adolescence also cause a reduction in pulmonary function (16). For example, Tsimoyianis and associates found that adolescent athletes exposed passively to cigarette smoke had nine times more pulmonary symptoms than did adolescents who had not been exposed (17). The other major concern associated with adolescent smoking is its affect on fetal growth and development. Maternal smoking is associated with a 30% decrease in fetal oxygen and with lower birth weight (18). According to a recent national survey, approximately 40% of first-time adolescent mothers smoked cigarettes during pregnancy (19).

The use of smokeless tobacco also has deleterious effects on health. These health problems include altered serum lipid levels, oral cancer, gingival recession, gingivitis, periodontal disease, and leukoplakia (20–22). Smokeless tobacco is also addictive and should not be considered a "safe" alternative to smoking.

JUSTIFICATION

How Can Tobacco Use By Adolescents Be Identified Accurately?

Screening for tobacco use can be accomplished either through direct questioning or through biochemical measurements. In a clinical setting, screening is almost always done through either a clinical interview or through a self report questionnaire. Among adolescents, smoking does not appear to have the same negative social stigma as do other health-risk behaviors, such as drinking and sexual behavior (23). In fact, recent data indicate that high school students associate certain cigarette product symbols with desirable personality traits, such as being "cool" and "interesting" (24). Although they sometimes tend to minimize tobacco use, adolescents are likely to be honest with their answers to questions regarding smoking. Pechacek and associates compared the results of self report questionnaires to biochemical tests of nicotine among 2,200 junior and senior high school students (23). Adolescents' self reports of smoking behaviors correlated well (r = .5–.7) with saliva testing and expired carbon monoxide. Adolescents older than age 13 were substantially more likely to report accurately compared to younger adolescents.

Biochemical tests have been developed which measure the three basic byproducts of tobacco—carbon monoxide in the blood or expired alveolar air, cotinine which is a primary metabolite of nicotine, and thiocyanate which is a detoxification product of hydrogen cyanide in tobacco smoke. Although tests of all three byproducts appear to provide reliable results, use of these tests has been limited to smoking research (8, 23–25).

What are the Most Effective Preventive Interventions for Adolescent Tobacco Use?

Preventive interventions directed at tobacco use among adolescents usually involve a primary strategy to keep adolescents from starting to smoke, and a secondary preventive strategy to identify smokers prior to habituation and involve them in a cessation program.

The majority of efforts at primary prevention of smoking have occurred through school health education. Early education strategies for smoking prevention were oriented toward teaching children about the long-term health problems associated with smoking (26, 27). Scare tactics were often employed whereby adolescents were provided with vivid details of adverse health consequences associated with smoking. These programs, which relied heavily on the theory that fear of consequences would help adolescents choose not to smoke, had relatively weak positive effects. Newer and more successful programs have been implemented that are oriented to the developmental needs of the adolescent. These programs emphasize the short-term physical and social consequences of smoking and the skills needed to avoid smoking initiation (26, 27). The roles of family and peers are also being incorporated into prevention programs, especially programs that emphasize social skills training (27). Developmentally oriented programs recognize the window of opportunity between initiation and habitual smoking, and they emphasize interventions that interrupt this progression (28, 29).

Review of research studies indicates that successful office-based intervention programs with adults incorporate repeated messages from both physician and nonphysician counselors. These programs have used audiovisual instruction and other methods of intervention, including counseling, self-help booklets, and nicotine chewing gum (30, 31). Physicians who briefly discuss smoking cessation, offer nicotine gum and/or set a quit date, and have follow-up appointments with patients can increase smoking cessation by two to seven times over those physicians who do not use such strategies (32, 33).

The National Cancer Institute (NCI) has developed a smoking cessation program for adults to be used by physicians in clinical settings (34). An adaptation of this program for children and adolescents has also been developed (35, 36). Results from controlled clinical trials with 700 physicians and 40,000 adult subjects using the NCI program suggest that physicians can influence patients' smoking habits by (1) asking about smoking at every opportunity; (2) advising all smokers to stop; (3) assisting patients with stop-smoking contracts, and self-help and motivating materials; (3) setting a quit date and prescribing nicotine gum; and (5) arranging follow-up visits to reinforce the intervention (34). Although a cessation strategy does appear effective in reducing smoking among adults, the NCI program has not been thoroughly studied among adolescents. In addition, the safety and efficacy of nicotine gum or the new transdermal nicotine patches for adolescents have not determined.

The most widely studied smoking prevention strategies for adolescents have been school and community-based interventions directed both at prevention of first use and at cessation. Results from a study by Hirschman and Leventhal suggest that, with as few as three health education sessions, the proportion of adolescents who progress from first use of cigarettes to more regular use can be decreased (29). Data from numerous studies indicate that school health education programs directed at helping adolescents develop skills to resist social pressures to smoke can generally reduce the onset of smoking by 50% (27–29, 37, 38). Although multiple health education sessions generally are not practical for the office setting, physicians and office staff can reinforce the social skills training learned in school. Preventive interventions reinforced in multiple settings have proven more effective in preventing smoking among adolescents than have strategies providing only school health education.

For example, Flynn and associates found a substantial reduction in smoking over 24 months among adolescents exposed to a targeted mass media intervention combined with health education (39). Results were not as good in adolescents whose only health education was through a school program. One reason for this combination strategy's effectiveness may be that health messages reinforced from a variety of creditable sources influence the adolescent's social norms which, in turn, influence behavior. Since possibly one-third of adolescents quit smoking on their own, social influences may be especially important early in a person's smoking history (40).

Physician messages that inform adolescents about the negative aspects of smoking might also help some youths quit. In one study, for example, Stone and Kristeller found that 80% of occasional smokers (those who smoke, but not daily) and 65% of daily smokers reported that they wanted to quit smoking (41). General health concerns were reported as the main reason for wanting to quit by 70% of occasional smokers and by 43% of those in the study who smoked daily.

CLINICAL APPLICATION

As described by the National Cancer Institute, physicians can play a significant role in preventive tobacco use among adolescents. Recommendations include the following (35, 36):

1. Provide anticipatory guidance to adolescents who do not use to-bacco products to prepare them for the social pressures they will face from peers and other environmental sources.
2. Ask adolescents at every visit whether they or any of their friends smoke or use chewing tobacco.
3. Advise adolescents who use tobacco products that nicotine is addictive and that it is easier to stop use now before it becomes a habit. This advise should include a discussion of the immediate effects of tobacco, such as odor on clothes and on the breath, stains on fingers and teeth, and reduced exercise performance.
4. Help adolescents stop smoking by:

- Developing a mutual understanding of the problem.

- Developing a stop-smoking plan that is realistic.

- Developing a stop-date.

- Identifying barriers to cessation and using role playing to identify ways to overcome these barriers.

- Providing self-help written material and telling adolescents about self-help groups.

5. Arranging follow-up visits to review progress.

In addition to these recommendations from the NCI, physicians can also discuss with parents the influence their own smoking has on their children. Parents who smoke should be encouraged to stop, and they should be provided with help in developing a cessation plan.

REFERENCES

1. Moss AJ, Allen KF, Giovino GA, Mills SL. Recent trends in adolescent smoking, smoking-uptake correlates, and expectations about the future. Advance data from vital and health statistics; 221. Hyattsville, MD: National Center for Health Statistics, 1992.
2. Allen KF, Moss AJ, Giovino GA, Shopland DR, Pierce JP. Teenage tobacco use: data estimates from the Teenage Attitudes and Practices Survey, United States, 1989. Advance data from vital and health statistics; 224. Hyattsville, MD: National Center for Health Statistics, 1992.
3. Centers for Disease Control. Prevalence of oral lesions and smokeless tobacco use in Northern Plains Indians. MMWR 1988;37:608–611.

4. Johnston LD, O'Malley PM, Bachman JG. National Trends in Drug Use and Related Factors Among American High School Students and Young Americans. 1975–1986. DHHS Publication No. (ADM) 87–1535. Washington, DC: US Government Printing Office, 1987.

5. US Department of Health and Human Services. Reducing the Health Consequences of Smoking: 25 Years of Progress: A Report of the Surgeon General, 1989. DHHS Publication No. (CDC) 89–8411. Washington, DC: US Government Printing Office, 1989.

6. Escobedo LG, Anda RF, Smith PF, Remington PL, Mast EE. Sociodemographic characteristics of cigarette smoking initiation in the United States. JAMA 1990; 264:1550–1555.

7. Baugh JG, Hunter SM, Webber LS, Berenson GS. Developmental trends of first cigarette smoking experience in children: the Bogalusa Heart Study. Am J Public Health 1982;72:1161–1164.

8. Haley NJ, Axelrod CM, Tilton KA. Validation of self-reported smoking behavior: biochemical analysis of cotinine and thiocyanate. Am J Public Health 1983;73:1204–1207.

9. Kandel DB, Davies M, Karus D, Yamaguchi K. The consequences in young adulthood of adolescent drug involvement. Arch Gen Psychiatry 1986;43:746–754.

10. Kandel DB, Logan JA. Patterns of drug use from adolescence to young adulthood: I. Periods of risk for initiation, continued use, and discontinuation. Am J Public Health 1984;74:660–666.

11. Raveis VH, Kandel DB. Changes in drug behavior from the middle to the late twenties: initiation, persistence, and cessation of use. Am J Public Health 1987;77:607–611.

12. Goldbaum GM, Kendrick JS, Hogelin GC, Gentry EM, and Behavioral Risk Factors Surveys Group. The relative impact of smoking and oral contraceptive use on women in the United States. JAMA 1987;258:1339–1342.

13. Loeb LA, Ernster VL, Warner KE, et al. Smoking and lung cancer: an overview. Cancer Res 1984;44:5940–5958.

14. Craig WY, Palomaki GE, Johnson AM, Haddow JE. Cigarette smoking-associated changes in blood lipid levels in the 8- to 19-year-old age group: a meta-analysis. Pediatrics 1990;85:155–158.

15. Webber LS, Hunter SM, Baugh JG, et al. The interaction of cigarette smoking, oral contraceptive use, and cardiovascular risk factor variables in children: The Bogalusa Heart Study. Am J Public Health 1982;72:266–274.

16. Tager IB, Muncz A, Rosener B, et al. Longitudinal analysis of the effects of cigarettes smoking in children. Chest 1984;85(suppl):8s.

17. Tsimoyianis GV, Jacobson MS, Feldman JG, et al. Reduction in pulmonary function and increased frequency of cough associated with passive smoking in teenage athletes. Pediatrics 1987;80:32–36.

18. Zuckerman B. Drug-exposed infants: understanding the medical risk. Future of Children 1991;1:26–35.

19. Abma JC, Mott FL. Substance use and prenatal care during pregnancy among young women. Fam Plann Perspect 1991;23:117–122.

20. US Department of Health and Human Services. The Health Consequences of Using Smokeless Tobacco, A Report of the Advisory Committee to the Surgeon General. NIH Publication No. 86–2874. Washington, DC: US Government Printing Office, 1986.

21. Feldman J, Shenker IR, Etzel RA, et al. Passive smoking alters lipid profiles in adolescents. Pediatrics 1991;88:259–264.

22. Consensus Conference. Health applications of smokeless tobacco use. JAMA 1986;255:1045–1048.

23. Pechacek TF, Murray DM, Luepker RV, Mittelmark MB, Johnson CA, Shutz JM. Measurement of adolescent smoking behavior: rationale and methods. J Behav Med 1984;7:123–140.

24. DiFranza JR, Richards JW, Paulman PM, et al. RJR Nabisco's cartoon camel promotes camel cigarettes to children. JAMA 1991;266:3149–3153.

25. Luepker RV, Pechacek TF, Murray DM, Johnson CA, Hund F, Jacobs DR. Saliva thiocyanate: a chemical indicator of cigarette smoking in adolescents. Am J Public Health 1981;71:1320–1324.

26. Miller SK, Slap GB. Adolescent smoking: a review of prevalence and prevention. J Adolesc Health Care 1989;10:129–135.

27. Murray DM, Luepker RV, Johnson CA, Mittelmark MB. The prevention of cigarette smoking in children: a comparison of four strategies. J Appl Soc Psychol 1984;14:274–288.

28. Best JA, Thomson SJ, Santi SM, Smith EA, Brown S. Preventing cigarette smoking among school children. Annu Rev Public Health 1988;9:161–201.

29. Hirschman RS, Leventhal H. Preventing smoking behavior in school children: an initial test of a cognitive-development program. J Appl Soc Psychol 1989;19:559–583.

30. Kottke TE, Battista RN, DeFriese GH, Brekke ML. Attributes of successful smoking cessation interventions in medical practice: a meta-analysis of 39 controlled trials. JAMA 1988;259:2882–2889.

31. Ockene JK. Physician-delivered interventions for smoking cessation: strategies for increasing effectiveness. Prev Med 1987;16:723–737.

32. Cohen SJ, Stookey GK, Katz BP, Drook CA, Smith DM. Encouraging primary care physicians to help smokers quit. Ann Intern Med 1989;110:648–652.

33. Lindsay EA, Wilson DM, Best JA, et al. A randomized trial of physician training for smoking cessation. Am J Health Promotion 1989;3:11–18.

34. Glynn TJ, Manley MW. How to Help Your Patient Stop Smoking: A National Cancer Institute Manual for Physicians. DHHS Publication No. 90–3064. Washington, DC: US Government Printing Office, 1990.

35. Clinical Interventions to Prevent Tobacco Use by Children and Adolescents: A Supplement to How to Help Your Patients Stop Smoking: A National Cancer Institute Manual for Physicians. DHHS Publication No. 90–3064. Washington, DC: US Government Printing Office, 1990.

36. Epps RP, Manley MW. A physician's guide to preventing tobacco use during childhood and adolescence. Pediatrics 1991;88:140–144.

37. Battjes RJ. Prevention of adolescent drug abuse. Inter J Addict 1985;20:1113–1134.

38. Flay B. Psychosocial approaches to smoking prevention: a review of findings. Health Psychol 1985;4:449–488.

39. Flynn BS, Worden JK, Secker-Walker RH, Badger GJ, Geller BM, Costanza MC. Prevention of cigarette smoking through mass media interventions and school programs. Am J Public Health 1992;82:827–834.

40. Hansen WB, Collins LM, Johnson CA, Graham JW. Self-initiated smoking cessation among high school students. Addict Behav 1985;10:265–271.

41. Stone SL, Kristeller JL. Attitudes of adolescents toward smoking cessation. Am J Prev Med 1992;8:221–225.

CHAPTER 11

Rationale and Recommendations: Use of Alcohol, Other Drugs, and Anabolic Steroids

PREVENTION STRATEGY

GAPS recommends a multiphasic strategy to prevent the use and abuse of alcohol, other psychoactive drugs, and anabolic steroids. This strategy involves (1) general health guidance to all parents regarding the need for them to monitor their adolescent's social and recreational activities for alcohol and drug use; (2) general health guidance to all adolescents, which includes information on the hazards of using alcohol, other psychoactive drugs, and anabolic steroids; and (3) screening and early intervention. In order to promote open and honest disclosure of information, screening should be performed in a confidential manner. Routine use of urine toxicology to screen for drug use is not recommended. Because health-risk behaviors frequently occur together, physicians should be especially alert to tobacco use and involvement in sexual behavior among adolescents who use alcohol and other drugs. Guidelines for health guidance directed at preventing substance use are included in Recommendation 10; screening for substance use is included in Recommendation 15.

DISCUSSION

The terminology used to describe alcohol and drug use is controversial and confusing (1). Because alcohol use and psychoactive drug use among adolescents are illegal, some health professionals consider any use of these substances as abuse. This legal framework, however, does not take into account the experimental and social nature of most alcohol and drug use, and it identifies all users as offenders. Based on a developmental framework, other health professionals differentiate among the following types of use: (1) casual, experimental, or recreational use, which is driven by social factors and occurs within a context of relatively healthy psychosocial adjustment; (2) abuse, which is associated with underlying emotional distress, involves heavy and multiple drug use, and has adverse consequences for interpersonal relationships and social functioning; and (3) physical or psychological dependency.

Alcohol

Alcohol remains the most widely used psychoactive substance among adolescents. Approximately 50% of all adolescents age 12–17, and 90% of high school seniors, have used alcohol at least once in their lives. Sixty percent of seniors are current users (2, 3). Among high school seniors who have used alcohol, 11% reported they first tried alcohol in the 6th grade (2). However, even more significant than the number of adolescents who have had a drink of alcohol are data indicating the intensity or frequency of use. Results of national surveys indicate that 30–44% of high school seniors, 23–36% of 10th graders, and over 10% of 8th graders report a recent episode of binge drinking, defined as having five or more drinks at one time (1, 2). These rates are somewhat greater for males than for females. A recent study of students attending colleges in the Northeast revealed that approximately 31% of males and 14% of females were frequent or heavy users of alcohol (4). More than half of college males (56%) and over one third of females (35%) had a recent episode of binge drinking.

Other Psychoactive Drugs

Some progress has been made to reduce psychoactive drug use among adolescents. Between 1980 and 1990, the rate of high school seniors who used a psychoactive drug (other than alcohol) declined from 53% to 29% (2). In general, students today better understand the harmful effects of drugs and are less tolerant toward their use. Serious problems, however, still remain. Approximately 40% of high school seniors have used marijuana; 14–18% are current users of marijuana; and another 2% report using marijuana daily (2, 3). Of all adolescents age 12–17, 15% have used marijuana, 8% have used an inhalant psychoactive substance, 3–6% have used cocaine, and 3% have used a hallucinogen. Approximately 2% of adolescents are current users of cocaine.

Initiation of marijuana (and also inhalants) increases dramatically between 6th and 9th grades, while first use of cocaine (and hallucinogens) occurs somewhat later, after the 9th grade (2). At all ages, males are more likely than females to use psychoactive drugs.

Anabolic Steroids

The use of anabolic steroids appears to be a growing problem among adolescents. From 5–11% of high school students have used anabolic steroids (5–9). Males use steroids two to seven times more frequently than do females; use among athletes is twice that of non-athletes. Approximately 20% of intercollegiate athletes use anabolic steroids, compared to approximately 1% of non-athletes (10). Athletes may abuse a variety of drugs, as well as anabolic steroids, in order to enhance their performance. For example, Krowchuk and associates found that almost 2% of high school athletes used amphetamines, 35% used proteins, and 33% used vitamins to enhance their performance (7). Twenty-five percent of this sample believed it was appropriate to use anabolic steroids to enhance performance, while 12% supported amphetamine use, and another 75% believed that protein and vitamin supplements were appropriate.

Consequences of Substance Use and the Relationship Between Use and Other Health Behaviors

Prevalence rates fail to reflect adequately the magnitude of adolescent health problems associated with alcohol and drug use. Many adolescents who drink or use psychoactive drugs place themselves and others at high risk for death and serious injury. For example, 10–20% of adolescents report that they drove a motor vehicle after using alcohol or other drugs, while 10–15% report substance use while swimming or boating (4, 11–14). In addition, 35–50% of adolescents report they rode recently with a driver who had consumed two or more drinks prior to driving. With such widespread use, especially in situations where impaired judgment is hazardous, it is not surprising that alcohol and other substance use is associated with the leading causes of death for adolescents. These causes include motor vehicle crashes, interpersonal violence, and suicide.

Although legislation that increased the minimum drinking age reduced motor vehicle fatalities, the leading cause of death in adolescence remains motor vehicle crashes, half of which are related to use of alcohol by adolescent drivers (15, 16). Overall, approximately 20% of deaths among adolescents age 15–20 are from alcohol-related car crashes (1, 17). In addition, alcohol is associated with 50% of homicide deaths, 30% of suicides, and 24% of fatal pedestrian or bicycle accidents among adolescents (18). A more complete discussion of the association between substance use and injuries is found in Chapter 4.

Results from longitudinal studies demonstrate a sequence or pattern of substance use. Usually, adolescents progress from using cigarettes to alcohol, to marijuana, and then to other illicit drugs (19, 20). Because of this progression, cigarettes and alcohol are considered "gateway" drugs. Although most adolescents who use marijuana and other psychoactive drugs have previously used alcohol and cigarettes, the reverse is not true (19, 20).

Adolescent alcohol and psychoactive drug use, especially among those in whom use shows an abusive pattern, is frequently associated with other health-risk behaviors. For example, among high school seniors, those who use marijuana are 80% more likely than non-users to have been injured in an automobile accident, fight, or assault during the past year (2). Among college students, binge drinking is associated with higher rates of unplanned sexual activity, missing classes, academic difficulties, and trouble with the police (4). Substance use is also associated with early initiation of sexual activity and unsafe sexual practices (21). Substance use lowers sexual inhibitions and may increase the risk for unintended pregnancies and sexually transmissible diseases (including HIV infection), especially when sex is exchanged for drugs. Adolescents who abuse substances tend to have multiple sexual contacts and not to use condoms (22). The risk of transmission of HIV infection also increases when the substances used are intravenous drugs.

Alcohol and psychoactive drug abuse among adolescents frequently occurs concomitantly with other mental disorders, including depression (23–25), suicide ideation, and suicide behavior (26, 27). For example, Garrison and associates studied data from a sample of over 3,600 high school students to determine the association between suicidal behavior (e.g., thoughts, plans, and attempts requiring medical care) and involvement in alcohol and other drugs (27). After controlling for race and gender, adolescents who reported heavy use of any substance had, in general, a two to three times increased risk for each category of suicidal behavior when compared to nonsubstance-using adolescents.

Alcohol, drug, and steroid use affect the physical and psychological health of adolescents in other ways as well. For example, research on marijuana indicates that use may decrease cognitive functioning (28) and may adversely affect the lung (29–31). Cocaine can cause cardiac arrhythmias that lead to sudden death (32–34).

Not only does abuse of alcohol and other drugs have immediate effects, adolescent onset abuse is also associated with adverse health and social consequences during later years (35). Most adults who abuse alcohol or illegal drugs began their use during adolescence (19). Substance abuse among adults is also associated with various psychosocial morbidities, such as poor interpersonal relationships (including marriage) and vocational difficulties

(35). Chronic use of alcohol is the principal contributor to cirrhosis of the liver, and can cause vascular and neurological disease (36).

Alcohol and drug use during pregnancy has profound effects on the developing fetus. Fetal alcohol syndrome (FAS), caused by chronic and excessive use of alcohol during pregnancy, and prenatal use of cocaine and other psychoactive drugs are associated with learning disabilities, attention deficit disorder, antisocial behavior, failure to grow, and abnormalities of the heart, kidneys, and skeletal system (37, 38).

FAS is the leading known cause of mental retardation in the United States. As of 1987, the estimated cost for health problems related to fetal alcohol syndrome (including growth retardation, organic anomalies requiring surgical repair, treatment of sensorineural problems, and mental retardation) was $321 million (38). Cocaine use during pregnancy also can cause severe problems, including spontaneous abortions (37, 39), and neurobehavioral and immune system abnormalities among affected newborns. Other substances (marijuana, methamphetamines, opiates, and PCP) also have negative and long lasting effects on the health of fetuses (37, 39). Results from a recent national survey indicate that approximately 6% of first-time mothers under the age of 20 drank alcohol during pregnancy, and approximately 19% smoked marijuana (40).

Inappropriate use of anabolic steroids can also have various adverse health consequences. Excessive use of steroids affect hepatic, gonadal, and psychological function, as well as serum lipids and blood pressure (41). Recent deaths of professional athletes from suicide and cancer have brought national attention to the health hazards of steroid use.

Justification

How Can Alcohol and Other Drug Use Among Adolescents Be Best Identified?

In order to obtain accurate information about substance use, adolescents and health professionals generally concur that screening should be done in the privacy of the physician-adolescent relationship (42–44). If ensured that their information will remain confidential, adolescents appear willing to provide reliable historical information about their substance use. For example, in one study of substance-abusing adolescents, approximately 80% of subjects reported that they would discuss their drug use with their primary physician, if the information remained confidential (42). Similar results were obtained from nonsubstance-abusing adolescents seen in a suburban clinic (43). Needle and associates assessed the reliability of high school students' answers to questions about substance use (45). Responses to questions asked at school and again at home demonstrated a test/retest reliability for reported alcohol or substance use of approximately 91%. In addition, researchers found no positive responses to use of a fictitious drug.

Currently, most physicians do not routinely screen adolescents for use of alcohol or other drugs (42, 46). Predictably, adolescent substance use is underdetected in the clinical setting. For example, Duggan and associates found that physicians identified from face-to-face interviews only 1 in 22 adolescents who were identified from self-report measures as using drugs (47). Singer and associates found that physicians identified only 1 in 4 adolescents who screened positive for alcohol use on a standard questionnaire (48). A number of questionnaires have been developed and tested that aid in the screening of adolescents for their risk of substance use (49, 50). Health professionals generally agree, however, that although questionnaires may promote screening for sensitive information, they should not substitute for a face-to-face interview.

Klitzner and Schonberg propose that questionnaires are appropriate under certain situations (51): (1) when providers want to screen adolescents not suspected as current users for health risks that could result from future use; (2) when providers suspect that adolescents are not providing truthful information because the clinical interview is too threatening; and (3) when providers think that direct questioning would alienate adolescents or their parents. An additional method of screening adolescents for alcohol and drug use is through computer-assisted health interviews, which have the additional benefit of providing personalized health education (52, 53). In one study, Paperny and associates found that a computer interview was preferred by adolescents over a clinical interview for obtaining sensitive information (52). Automated screening provided a greater positive response rate for health-risk behaviors, especially for high levels of alcohol or marijuana use.

Among adolescents who do use alcohol or other drugs, primary care physicians are faced with making a distinction between low-intensity use, which is more experimental in nature, and abuse or dependency. Suspicion of abuse can be obtained from the results of a relatively brief clinical interview. For example, Halikas found that responses to six key clinical screening questions (see Clinical Application section) distinguished adolescents who used alcohol and other substances in a more social or experimental fashion from those who abused substances (54, 55). Among groups of substance-abusing adolescents, 88–94% gave a positive response to at least one question, while among adolescents without abuse only 6–15% gave a positive response.

Once substance abuse is suspected, a more presumptive definitive diagnosis can be obtained from standardized questionnaires (47). Written questionnaires have the advantage over in-depth clinical interviews of reducing rater bias and taking less of the health provider's time. Comprehensive questionnaires have also been developed recently to assess the range of health and social problems experienced by adolescents who abuse alcohol and other drugs (56–59). Responses to these inventories provide a comprehensive functional assessment that is useful in planning a management strategy.

Various laboratory techniques are available to identify selective psychoactive substances in the urine. The routine use of urine testing to initially identify adolescent drug use, especially when the adolescent is unaware of the test, is controversial and of questionable value (60–62). GAPS does not recommend routine urine testing as an initial screening procedure for several reasons: (1) urine testing is expensive; (2) it has questionable validity and reliability unless performed under conditions that are rigorously controlled and monitored, from the initial collection of urine through laboratory testing; and (3) it may appear to adolescents as punitive and as an invasion of privacy and, therefore, undermine the development of an open, honest adolescent-physician relationship. In circumstances other than routine screening, the health benefit of testing can outweigh the ethical and practical liabilities. For example, urine testing might be appropriate to monitor adolescents who have been through initial drug abuse treatment and are involved in an aftercare program.

Are Clinical Interventions Effective in Preventing or Reducing Adolescents' Use of Alcohol, Drugs, and Steroids?

Justification to support the utility of health guidance for the prevention of alcohol and drug use comes from the belief that health messages provided by physicians, as sources of creditable information, can affect behavioral change in drinking and other drug use. Within clinical settings, adolescents receive personalized, face-to-face interactions that may have a greater impact than preventive interventions provided in group settings or through the mass media. Furthermore, health messages provided by primary practitioners reinforce information already received from teachers, parents, and other adults. Reinforcement of these messages in various settings has a greater effect on behavioral change than do preventive interventions delivered by only one source (63).

For example, Pentz and associates developed and tested a community-based primary prevention program directed toward reducing drug and alcohol use among adolescents, as well as reducing other risk factors associated with cardiovascular disease (63, 64). The program used three components: (1) school health education, (2) mass media public information, and (3) help for parents to improve their own personal health behaviors. A special analysis of data from this program revealed that adding the parent component produced a greater reduction of heavy alcohol and marijuana use than when the school and mass media components were used alone (63). Overall, the preventive intervention effectively reduced adolescent alcohol and substance use by 5.2% for monthly drunkenness and 2.9% for weekly use of marijuana. Other studies have also shown that combining a mass media approach with a school health education strategy increases the effectiveness of the intervention (65).

In general, health education is most effective at changing behaviors when it is oriented toward helping adolescents develop social skills to resist peer pressure, reshape attitudes toward drug use, and learn more healthy ways to cope with stress (66, 67). Effective health education also incorporates family training (68, 69). Those interventions that offer information only (70), offer graphic information on consequences of substance use (71), or provide punitive behavior modification (72) have questionable behavioral results. For example, Goldberg and associates studied the effects of two types of health education on adolescent football players' attitudes toward steroid use (71). In contrast to adolescents who received a "scare tactics" intervention, adolescents who received a "balanced" health education program developed greater negative attitudes toward steroid use.

Although the effectiveness of brief office counseling directed at reducing low-frequency substance use among adolescents has not been studied, there is some evidence that this strategy has been effective with adults. For example, results of studies by Moore and associates using an inpatient population and Logsdon and associates using an outpatient population suggest that a brief physician intervention can reduce alcohol use among adults (73, 74).

CLINICAL INTERVENTION

GAPS recommends both primary and secondary preventive strategies to reduce adolescents' use of alcohol, drugs, and steroids. The primary prevention strategy calls for physicians to provide health guidance to all adolescents, with instruction on the dangers of substance use and ways to refrain from use. The intent of this strategy is to reinforce health messages received in school and in the home. This strategy is complemented by recommendations to counsel parents to monitor adolescents' social behaviors, especially when the use of psychoactive substances and impaired judgment may be harmful.

GAPS also recommends a secondary preventive intervention in which physicians screen adolescents for use of alcohol and other drugs and, if use is identified, either provide brief counseling or refer the adolescent for more in-depth assessment and treatment. Although most adolescents will experiment with psychoactive substances, the majority of them are not at high risk for abuse or adverse health outcomes. Substance use in any of the following circumstances, however, should be considered a problem that necessitates an in-depth evaluation (75):

1. Use of substances that are inherently dangerous (e.g., crack cocaine).
2. Use of alcohol or other drugs by preadolescents.
3. Use of alcohol or other drugs in inappropriate settings (e.g., while driving or in school).
4. Use of alcohol or drugs when there are clear signs of tolerance, withdrawal, or dependence.

GAPS suggests that previsit questionnaires only be used to determine risk for substance use, while direct questioning of actual use be performed during a clinical interview. Once use is identified, a positive response to any of the following questions should alert the health provider to possible abuse and prompt a referral (54, 55):

1. Does the adolescent ever use drugs when alone?
2. Does the adolescent ever use alcohol when alone?
3. Does the adolescent ever get drunk or high at social events or have friends who do?
4. Does the adolescent ever consume alcohol on school grounds?
5. Does the adolescent ever miss school because of drinking or hangovers?
6. When truant, does the adolescent ever go drinking or get high on drugs?

Standardized questionnaires can be used to further define the substance use pattern. Information from the clinical interview, and possibly the written questionnaire, should be used to determine the nature of substance use and whether the adolescent is at risk for adverse health consequences. The physical examination has only limited value in assessing adolescent alcohol and drug use. Regardless of the substance use pattern, physicians should determine whether the adolescent is involved in other health-risk behaviors, such as smoking and sexual behaviors that might lead to unintended pregnancy or STD, including HIV infection. If other health-risk behaviors are identified, a strategy to address these problems should be included in a management plan.

All adolescent males who participate in high school athletic programs should be asked about their knowledge and use of anabolic steroids. Special attention should be given to those who participate in sports that require weight and strength, such as football, track and field, and weightlifting.

REFERENCES

1. US Congress, Office of Technology Assessment. Adolescent Health-Volume II: Background and the Effectiveness of Selected Prevention and Treatment Services. OTA-H-466. Washington, DC: US Government Printing Office, 1991: 499–578.

2. Johnston LD, O'Malley PM, Bachman JG. Drug Use Among American High School Seniors, College Students and Young Adults, 1975–1990. Volume I: High School Seniors. DHHS Publication No. (ADM) 91–1813. Rockville, MD: National Institute on Drug Abuse, 1991.

3. Centers for Disease Control. Alcohol and other drug use among high school students—United States, 1990. MMWR 1991;40:776–777, 783–784.

4. Wechsler H, Isaac N: "Binge" drinkers at Massachusetts colleges. Prevalence, drinking style, time trends, and associated problems. JAMA 1992;267:2929–2931.

5. Buckley WE, Yasalis CE, Friedl KE, et al. Estimated prevalence of anabolic steroid use among male high school seniors. JAMA 1988;260:3441–3445.

6. Johnson MD, Jay MS, Shoup B, Rickert VI. Anabolic steroid use by male adolescents. Pediatrics 1989;83:921–924.

7. Krowchuk DP, Anglin TM, Goodfellow DB, Stancin T, Williams P, Zimet GD. High school athletes and the use of ergogenic aids. Am J Dis Child 1989;143:486–489.

8. Terney R, McLain L. The use of anabolic steroids in high school students. Am J Dis Child 1990;144:99–103.

9. Komoroski EM, Richert VI. Adolescent body image and attitudes to anabolic steroid use. Am J Dis Child 1992;146:823–828.

10. Dezelsky T, Toohey J, Shaw R. Non-medical drug use behavior in five US universities: a 15-year study. Bull Narc 1985;37:49–53.

11. Centers for Disease Control. Factors potentially associated with reductions in alcohol-related traffic fatalities—United States, 1990 and 1991. MMWR 1992;41:893–899.

12. American School Health Association. The National Adolescent Student Health Survey: A Report on the Health of America's Youth. Oakland, CA: Third Party Publishing Co, 1989.

13. Klepp KI, Perry CL, Jacobs DR. Etiology of drinking and driving among adolescents: implications for primary prevention. Health Educ Q 1991;18:415–427.

14. Williams AF, Lund AK, Preusser DF. Drinking and driving among high school students. Inter J Addict 1986;21:643–655.

15. Decker M, Graitcar P, Schaffner W. Reduction in motor vehicle fatalities associated with an increased minimum drinking age. JAMA 1988;260:3604–3610.

16. Centers for Disease Control. Quarterly table reporting alcohol involvement in fatal motor vehicle crashes. MMWR 1991;40:647.

17. Centers for Disease Control. Childhood injuries in the United States. Am J Dis Child 1990;144:646–727.

18. US Public Health Service. Health United States 1989 and Prevention Profile. Washington, DC: US Department of Health and Human Services, 1990.

19. Kandel DB, Logan JA. Patterns of drug use from adolescence to young adulthood: I. Periods of risk for initiation, continued use, and discontinuation. Am J Pub Health 1984;74:660–666.

20. Kandel D. Stages in adolescent involvement in drug use. Science 1974;190:912–914.

21. Zabin LS, Hardy JB, Smith EA, Hirsch MB. Substance use and its relation to sexual activity among inner-city adolescents. J Adolesc Health Care 1986;7:320–331.

22. Fullilove RE, Fullilove MT, Bowser BP, Gross SA. Risk of sexually transmitted disease among black adolescent crack users in Oakland and San Francisco, CA. JAMA 1990;263:851–855.

23. Kaplan SL, Landa B, Weinhold C, Shenker IR. Adverse health behaviors and depressive symptomatology in adolescents. J Am Acad Child Psychiatry 1984;23:595–601.

24. Deykin EY, Levy JC, Wells V. Adolescent depression, alcohol and drug abuse. Am J Public Health 1986;76:178–182.

25. Regier DA, Farmer ME, Rae DS, et al. Comorbidity of mental disorders with alcohol and other drug abuse: results from the Epidemiologic Catchment Area Study. JAMA 1990; 264:2511–2518.

26. Crumley FE. Substance abuse and adolescent suicidal behavior. JAMA 1990;263:3051–3056.

27. Garrison CZ, McKeown RE, Valois RF, Vincent ML. Aggression, substance use, and suicidal behaviors in high school students. Am J Public Health 1993;83:179–184.

28. Schwartz RH, Gruenewald PJ, Klitzner M, Fedio P. Short-term memory impairment in cannabis-dependent adolescents. Am J Dis Child 1989;143:1214–1219.

29. Bloom JW, Kaltenborn WT, Paoletti P, Camilli A, Lebowitz MD. Respiratory effects of non-tobacco cigarettes. Br Med J 1987;295:1516–1518.

30. Tashkin DP. Pulmonary complications of smoked substance abuse. West J Med 1990;152:525–530.

31. Wu TC, Tashkin DP, Djahed B, Rose JE. Pulmonary hazards of smoking marijuana as compared with tobacco. N Engl J Med 1988;318:347–351.

32. Cregler LL, Mark H. Cardiovascular dangers of cocaine abuse. Am J Cardiol 1986;57:1185–1186.

33. Karch SB, Billingham ME. The pathophysiology and etiology of cocaine-induced heart disease. Arch Pathol Lab Med 1988;112:225–230.

34. Lathers CM, Tyan LSY, Spino MM, Agarwal I. Cocaine-induced seizures, arrhythmias and sudden death. J Clin Pharmacol 1988;28:584–593.

35. Kandel DB, Davies M, Karus D, Yamaguchi K. The consequences in young adulthood of adolescent drug involvement: an overview. Arch Gen Psychiatry 1986; 43:746–754.

36. Charness ME, Simon RP, Greenberg DA. Medical progress: ethanol and the nervous system. N Engl J Med 1989;321:442–454.

37. Dixon SD. Effects of transplacental exposure to cocaine and methamphetamine on the neonate. West J Med 1989;150:436–442.

38. Abel EL, Sokol RJ. Incidence of fetal alcohol syndrome and economic impact of FAS-related anomalies. Drug Alcohol Depend 1987;19:51–70.

39. Chasnoff IJ, Burns WJ, Schnoll SH, Burns KA. Cocaine use in pregnancy. N Engl J Med 1985;313:666–669.

40. Abma JC, Mott FL. Substance use and prenatal care during pregnancy among young women. Fam Plann Perspect 1991;23:117–122.

41. US General Accounting Office. Drug Misuse: Anabolic Steroids and Human Growth Hormone. Washington, DC: US General Accounting Office, 1989.

42. Friedman LS, Johnson B, Brett AS. Evaluation of substance-abusing adolescents by primary care physicians. J Adolesc Health Care 1990;11:227–230.

43. Marks A, Malizio J, Hoch J, Brody R, Fisher M. Assessment of health needs and willingness to utilize health care resources of adolescents in a suburban population. J Pediatr 1983;102:456–460.

44. Malvin JH, Moskowitz JM. Anonymous versus identifiable self-reports of adolescent drug attitudes, intentions, and use. Pub Opin Q 1983;47:557–566.

45. Needle R, McCubbin H, Lorence J, Hochhauser M. Reliability and validity of adolescent self-reported drug use in a family-based study: a methodological report. Inter J Addict 1983;18:901–912.

46. Greer SW, Bauchner H, Zuckerman B. Pediatricians' knowledge and practices regarding parental use of alcohol. Am J Dis Child 1990;144:1234–1237.

47. Duggan AK, Adger H, McDonald EM, Stokes EJ, Moore R. Detection of alcoholism in hospitalized children and their families. Am J Dis Child 1991;145:613–617.

48. Singer MI, Petchen MK, Anglin J. Detection of adolescent substance abuse in a pediatric outpatient department: a double-blind study. J Pediatr 1987;11:938–941.

49. Klitzner M, Schwartz RH, Grunewald P, Blasinsky M. Screening for risk factors for adolescent alcohol and drug use. Am J Dis Child 1987;141:45–49.

50. Petchers MK, Singer MI, Angelotta JW. Revalidation and expansion of an adolescent substance abuse screening measure. J Dev Behav Pediatr 1988;9:25–29.

51. Klitzner M, Schonberg SK. Concerns regarding the indirect assessment for drug abuse among adolescents. J Dev Behav Pediatr 1988;9:30–31.

52. Paperny DM, Aono JY, Lehman RM, Hammer SL, Risser J. Computer-assisted detection and intervention in adolescent high-risk health behaviors. J Pediatr 1990;116:456–462.

53. Millstein SG, Irwin CD. Acceptability of computer-acquired sexual histories in adolescent girls. J Pediatr 1983;103:815–819.

54. Halikas J. Substance abuse in children and adolescents. In: Garfinkel B, Carlson G, Weller E, eds. Textbook of Child and Adolescent Psychiatry. WB Saunders Co, 1990:210–234.

55. Halikas JA, Lyttle M, Morse C, Hoffman R. Proposed criteria for the diagnosis of alcohol abuse in adolescence. Compr Psychiatry 1984;25:581–585.

56. Henly GA, Winters KC. Development of problem severity scales for the assessment of adolescent alcohol and drug abuse. Inter J Addict 1988;23:65–85.

57. Henly GA, Winters KC. Development of psychosocial scales for the assessment of adolescent alcohol and drug abuse. Inter J Addict 1989;24:973–1001.

58. National Institute on Drug Abuse. The Adolescent Assessment/Referral System Manual. DHHS Publication No. (ADM) 91–1735. Washington, DC: Alcohol, Drug Abuse, and Mental Health Association, 1991.

59. Tarter RE, Hegedus AM. The Drug Use Screening Inventory: its application in the evaluation and treatment of alcohol and other drug abuse. Alcoh Health Res World 1991;15:65–75.

60. Grabowski J, Lasagna L. Screening for drug use: technical and social aspects. Issues Sci Tech 1987; Winter:36–45.

61. King NMP, Cross AW. Moral and legal issues in screening for drug use in adolescents. J Pediatr 1987;111:249–250.

62. Schwartz HR, Hayden GF, Riddile M. Laboratory detection of marijuana use: experience with a photometric immunoassay to measure urinary cannabinoids. Am J Dis Child 1985;139:1093–1096.

63. Pentz MA. Benefits of integrating strategies in different settings. In: Elster AB, Panzarine S, Holt K, eds. American Medical Association State of the Art Conference on Adolescent Health Promotion: Proceedings. McLean, VA: National Maternal and Child Health Clearinghouse, 1993.

64. Pentz MA, Johnson CA, Dwyer JH, et al. A comprehensive community approach to adolescent drug abuse prevention: effects on cardiovascular disease risk behaviors. Ann Med 1988;21:219–222.

65. Flynn BS, Worden JK, Secker-Walker RH, Badger GJ, Geller BM, Costanza MC. Prevention of cigarette smoking through mass media intervention and school programs. Am J Public Health 1992;82:827–834.

66. Botvin GJ. Prevention of adolescent substance abuse through the development of personal and social competence. In: Glynn T, Leukefeld G, Ludford J, eds. Preventing Adolescent Drug Abuse: Intervention Strategies. Rockville, MD: NIDA Research Monograph 47, 1984.

67. Botvin GJ. Substance abuse prevention research: recent developments and future directions. J Sch Health 1986;9:369–374.

68. Bry BH. Family-based approaches to reducing adolescent substance use: theories, techniques, and findings. NIDA Research Monograph Series 1988;77:39–68.

69. DeMarsh J, Kumpfer KL. Family-oriented interventions for the prevention of chemical dependency in children and adolescents. J Child Contemp Soc 1986;18:117–151.

70. Bruvold WH, Rundall TG. A meta-analysis and theoretical review of school-based tobacco and alcohol intervention programs. Psych Health 1988;2:53–78.

71. Goldberg L, Bents R, Bosworth E, Trevisian L, Elliot DL. Anabolic steroid education and adolescents: do scare tactics work? Pediatrics 1991;87:283–286.

72. Schwartz IM. Hospitalization of adolescents for psychiatric and substance abuse treatment. J Adolesc Health Care 1989;10:473–478.

73. Moore RD, Bone LR, Geller G, et al. Prevalence, detection, and treatment of alcoholism in hospitalized patients. JAMA 1989;261:403–407.

74. Logsdon DN, Lazaro CM, Meier RV. The feasibility of behavioral risk reduction in primary medical care. Am J Prev Med 1989;5:249–256.

75. Klitzner M, Fisher D, Stewart K, Gilbert S. Substance Abuse: Early Intervention for Adolescents. Washington, DC: Pacific Institute for Research and Evaluation, 1993.

CHAPTER 12

Rationale and Recommendation: Depression (Severe or Recurrent) and Suicide

PREVENTION STRATEGY

Because of the pervasive nature of mood disorders, all adolescents should be screened annually for signs and symptoms of recurrent or severe depression. Special attention should be directed at adolescents who are performing poorly in school, who use alcohol or drugs, or who have had a deteriorating relationship with parents or peers. Physicians should also screen adolescents annually to identify those at risk for suicide. Risk for suicide is not usually determined by any one single event, but rather by an accumulation of conditions, including family dysfunction, physical and sexual abuse, substance abuse, history of recurrent or severe depression, prior suicide attempt, and/or suicidal plans. Adolescents with a multiplicity of these factors should be interviewed further to determine their level of suicide risk. If suicidal intent is found, they should be referred for mental health evaluation or be hospitalized. Parents of adolescents at risk for suicide should be counseled to reduce access to firearms, weapons, or potentially lethal drugs within the home (GAPS Recommendation 4). Physician guidelines for depression and suicide are addressed in GAPS Recommendation 20.

DISCUSSION

Although adolescence is not as tumultuous as once believed, the complex physical, psychological, and social changes of this period present youth with major emotional challenges. Adolescents must cope with a variety of new stresses such as those associated with the physical changes of puberty, increasing academic demands, changing social roles, and opportunities for engaging in health-risk behaviors. Although most adolescents cope with

131

these stresses with minimal difficulty, some experience more serious emotional problems.

Zill and Schoenborn, using data from the 1988 National Health Interview Survey of Child Health, found that the proportion of children with emotional and behavioral problems rose from 5.3% at age 3–5, to 12.7% at age 6–11, to 18.5% at age 12–17 (1). Offer and associates, using a self-image questionnaire that measures various emotional domains, has found that approximately 20% of adolescents report feelings suggestive of emotional distress (2).

Results from a series of studies using data from the National Institute of Mental Health (NIMH) Epidemiological Catchment Area Program, a large household survey involving five U.S. communities, provide additional information about the epidemiology of adolescent emotional problems. In one study, Regier and associates found that 16.9% of youths 18–24 reported symptoms suggestive of a current mental health disorder, compared to 17.3% of people age 25–44 and 13.3% of those age 45–64 (3). The most frequent diagnoses for adolescents were mood disorders and use or abuse of alcohol and other drugs. In another study, Burke and associates compared birth cohorts over the past century and found a shift toward increased rates of major depressive and substance abuse disorders among youths age 15–19, compared to young adults (4). These and other results suggest that adolescence is a vulnerable period for the onset of various mental health problems, especially depression (4, 5).

DEPRESSION

Because transient fluctuations in mood can be associated with normal psychosocial development, depressive symptomatology is frequently reported by adolescents. For example, in a recent national study of 8th and 10th grade students (the National Adolescent Student Health Survey), 45% of adolescents reported difficulty coping with stressful situations at home and school, 24% frequently felt sad and hopeless, and 13% often felt they had nothing to look forward to (6). Although these rates did not vary by school grade, females reported greater levels of emotional distress than did males. Distinguishing transient, normal depressive mood swings from a more serious depressive disorder can be challenging. The latter usually includes a prolonged pessimism, while the former is short-lived and does not result in changes in school performance or family and peer relationships. This distinction is important and necessary because of the serious health consequences that can result from a depressive disorder.

Population estimates of major depressive disorder are usually made from results of self-report symptom checklists. A presumptive diagnosis of depression is made when a symptom profile conforms to standard psychiatric diagnostic criteria. Results from nonclinic populations indicate that, at any one time, from 3–5% of adolescents have persistent symptoms suggestive of a depressive disorder, and that possibly as many as 13–18% have had a major depressive episode at some time in their life (7–10). There does not appear to be consistency among study results regarding variation of depression by race or socioeconomic status (11). The risk of major depression is substantially greater, however, for adolescents whose parents have a mood disorder or suffer from alcoholism (11, 12). Genetic factors may also contribute to the risk for a depressive disorder (11).

Comparing the rate of recent feelings of sadness (approximately 24%) with the rate of current depression (3–5%) indicates that transient, depressed mood occurs five to eight times more frequently than does more serious depressive disorder. The large discrepancy between these two emotional states supports the notion that the psychological turmoil associated with adolescence leads to serious emotional difficulty in a relatively small proportion of youth.

Major depression can have significant immediate and long-term adverse consequences. Adolescents with a depressive disorder are more likely than others adolescents to use and abuse alcohol or other drugs, smoke cigarettes, attempt suicide, have academic difficulties, and exhibit other psychosocial difficulties and behavioral problems (8, 13, 14). The effects of adolescent depression frequently persist through later life. Adults who had a depressive disorder during adolescence are more likely to evince impaired psychological and social functioning and are more likely than other adults to have a mood disorder (15–17). A prior history of depressed mood is also associated with a increased risk for delinquent behavior and other health-risk behaviors (16).

SUICIDE

Suicide is the third leading cause of death for adolescents. The suicide rate for 15–19-year-olds has increased from 2.7 per 100,000 youths in 1950 to 11.3 per 100,000 youths in 1988 (18, 19). This increase has been especially large for white males, whose rates rose fourfold, from 3.7 per 100,000 in 1950 to 15 per 100,000 in 1980. A total of almost 2,000 adolescents age 15–19 and 3,500 youths 20–24 commit suicide each year. Suicide among youths 15–19 and 20–24 represents approximately 7% and 13% of all annual suicide deaths, respectively. Adolescent suicide is more common among males and youths who are white, Native American, homosexual, and those who are in juvenile correctional facilities (18–22). In an analysis of 12 studies, Schwartz and Whitaker computed a suicide rate among college students of 7.3 per 100,000 (23). This rate appeared to be approximately half the rate for comparable groups of nonstudents.

Experts estimate that suicide attempts occur up to 200 times more frequently than completed suicides (18). Adolescents who attempt suicide, in contrast to those who die from suicide, are more often female and Hispanic. The task of identifying adolescents at risk for suicide and studying the natural history of suicide ideation is complicated by two issues. First, most self-destructive behavior does not result in serious injury or hospitalization. Fewer than 25% of adolescents in a CDC survey who attempted suicide reported that they had received medical attention following the attempt (18). The second factor complicating the identification of suicidal risk is that from two to four times as many adolescents contemplate suicide as attempt suicide. Data from the CDC national Youth Risk Behavior Survey of almost 12,000 9th through 12th grade students indicate that 27% of adolescents (34% of females and 20.5% of males) had thought seriously about suicide during the previous 12 months (18). Sixteen percent of adolescents in this survey (20% of females and 12% of males) had made specific plans for suicide, and 8.3% had actually attempted suicide. These findings are similar to those of the National Adolescent Student Health Survey, in which 33% of adolescents reported that they had, at sometime in their lives, thought seriously about suicide, while 14% had previously attempted suicide (6). The results of other studies confirm the high rate of moderate to severe suicidal ideation among adolescents, especially females (24, 25).

Even though serious thoughts about suicide are relatively common, there have been few studies investigating the natural history of suicidal ideation among adolescents. After reviewing existing studies, Hawton concluded that while a majority of adolescents who attempt suicide improved emotionally over time, a substantial number continued to have major psychosocial difficulties (26). Hawton estimates that 25% of adolescents hospitalized for a suicide attempt have a history of a prior attempt. Viewing adolescents in a prospective manner, McIntire and associates estimated that at least 30% of adolescents with one suicide attempt will make a repeated attempt within a two-year period (27, 28). As reported by Shaffer and associates, follow-up studies suggest that from 1–9% of males and from less than 1% to 4% of females who attempt suicide eventually succeed in killing themselves (29).

For most adolescents who attempt suicide, a key mediating factor differentiating ideation from behavior appears to be the degree of hopelessness

resulting from chronic rather than acute events. Adolescents with more serious suicidal intent tend to have a history of emotional disorders and psychosocial difficulties, including depression, previous suicide attempts, alcohol or drug abuse, family dysfunction, conduct disorder, poor academic
performance, and maltreatment (13, 20, 24, 25, 30–37). In a large school-
based study, Garrison and associates found that major depression was more
common among adolescents with suicidal ideation and those who had attempted suicide than it was among nonsuicidal adolescents (24). Riggs and
associates, in a study of high school students, found that adolescents with a
history of sexual abuse were over three times more likely than other adolescents to have attempted suicide, and those with a history of physical abuse
were over five times more likely (37). Acute precipitating events, such as
family conflicts and social rejection are common, but not always present,
among adolescents who attempt suicide (29, 36, 38). There does appear to
be a group of suicidal adolescents who have difficulty with social adjustment
and respond to a precipitating stressful event with impulsive behavior (39).
These adolescents may also be influenced to suicide following television sto-
ries on suicide or following romantic pacts (40). Firearms are a major cause
of death among adolescents who commit suicide as a result of impulsive
behavior.

Brent and associates have presented impressive data suggesting that a
major component of the increase in adolescent suicide is the combination of
the availability of firearms and the use of alcohol (41, 42). In a large county-
wide study, suicide victims who used firearms were 4.9 times more likely to
have been drinking than were adolescents who used other ways to kill themselves (42). Community studies indicate that gun control may be effective in
lowering adolescent suicide. Supporting evidence for this view comes from
a study by Sloan and associates, who found that the suicide rate from firearms among adolescents in Vancouver, British Columbia—a city with a restrictive gun control law—is 10 times less than the rate in Seattle, a city with
a less restrictive gun control law (43). No studies, however, have investigated
the association between a clinical preventive strategy to reduce or limit the
availability of guns in the home and adolescent suicide.

JUSTIFICATION

How Can Primary Care Health Providers Best Identify Adolescents Who Have Severe or Recurrent Depression or Are at Risk for Suicide?

According to standard criteria, a diagnosis of a depressive disorder requires that adolescents have both a depressed or irritable mood and evidence

of diminished interest or pleasure in daily activities for at least a two-week period (44). They must also evince at least three of the following features: failure to gain expected weight, weight loss, or weight gain; insomnia or hypersomnia; psychomotor agitation or retardation; fatigue or loss of energy; feelings of worthlessness or excessive guilt; decreased concentration or indecisiveness; thoughts of death, suicidal ideation, or suicide attempt.

A variety of standardized questionnaires have been developed to assist in the diagnosis of adolescent depression (45, 46). Because of the risk of overdiagnosis, various panels and experts suggest that these instruments be used to verify a presumptive diagnosis of depression rather than to screen for depression among a general population (47, 48). As a general screening measure of persistent depressive symptomatology, expert opinion supports assessing for behavioral manifestations of disordered mood, such as a significant decline in academic performance. Other early signs include increased emotional distance from parents and friends and a loss of interest in regular social activities. Standardized questionnaires can be used to confirm a presumptive diagnosis of depression in an adolescent who exhibits these early signs.

No single factor predicts risk for suicide. Rather, for many adolescents risk appears to be a cumulative set of factors, including psychosocial variables, family function, past history of suicide behavior, depression, and alcohol or other drug use. For example, in a study of secondary school students, Lewinsohn and associates found that the probability of a past suicide attempt increased from 1% for adolescents with no or only one of a variety of risk factors, to 8% for those with three factors, to 29% for those with five factors, to 69% for those with seven or more factors (49). Although this relation was found for both genders, the association was greater for females than for males. For these adolescents, therefore, there appears to be a continuum of behavior from involvement in health-risk behaviors, to suicidal ideation, to serious suicidal intent and planning, and finally to actual self-destructive acts (24, 36). These youth often have a chronic history of emotional problems and depression. Screening for suicide risk for this group of adolescents, then, is best accomplished by assessing the cumulative factors that, taken together, may indicate a need for more in-depth assessment or referral. There are other adolescents at risk for suicide, however; they are impulsive, suffer from acute family or interpersonal crisis, and are without a chronic history of emotional or behavioral problems (39). For these youths, screening might be less effective. The relative size of these two groups of adolescents at risk for suicide is uncertain. The number of adolescents who are more deliberate in their actions, and for whom screening might be more successful, ranges from 40–80% (50, 51).

Adolescents with an emotional disorder are relatively common among populations seen in primary health care settings. The results of various studies suggest that from 6–12% of adolescents age 11–18 are identified by primary care physicians as having a psychosocial or mental health disorder (52–54). Schor reviewed five years of medical records of over 1,500 children enrolled in a managed care plan to determine the incidence of emotional disorders during childhood (53). The prevalence of psychological diagnosis increased for both genders during early adolescence compared to earlier ages, and then decreased with later adolescence. Approximately 10–12% of adolescents age 12–16 had a psychological diagnosis, such as depression or school adjustment problems. There is evidence, however, that adolescents with emotional health problems are underidentified by primary care providers.

For example, Hodgman and associates found that only 20% of pediatricians surveyed asked adolescents about suicidal ideation during a routine history (55). In a study involving children age 7–11, Costello and associates found that pediatricians underdiagnosed emotional and behavioral problems by approximately 50% (56). Although the physicians were highly specific with their diagnosis, their sensitivity for identifying children with emotional or behavioral problems was only 17%. In a recent study, Slap and associates presented questionnaires to 332 adolescents seen in an adolescent medicine clinic and found that 14.5% reported a previous suicide attempt (57). A review of the medical records of these 48 suicidal adolescents indicated, however, that only 16.7% were asked by their physician about self-destructive ideation or behavior. Somewhat better results were reported by Chang and associates, who found that primary care physicians identified psychological problems in 66% of children age 6–17 who had had at least one psychiatric diagnosis (58).

Does Early Identification Reduce the Risk of Adolescent Suicide?

Various efforts to prevent suicide by involving adolescents, regardless of risk, in school-based intervention programs, appear to have had little success (29, 59). GAPS efforts, therefore, are targeted toward secondary prevention, or the reduction in suicide risk among adolescents who are at greatest risk for self-destructive behavior.

Viewed from the perspective that suicide behavior is not a diagnosis, but rather the culmination of chronic conditions and acute psychosocial precipitants, the prevention of suicide through an office-based strategy is predominantly reliant on three strategies: (1) identification and management of the major determinant of self-destructive behavior, namely recurrent or severe depression; (2) identification of adolescents at risk for suicide and counseling to reduce availability in the home of firearms and potentially lethal medications, as well as informing adolescents about the availability of community crisis resources, such as suicide hotlines; and (3) identification and referral of adolescents who are in crisis and/or who have verbalized acute suicidal intent.

Support for these strategies comes predominantly from expert opinion. Although not studied in a clinical setting, it is anticipated that identification and management of adolescents with cumulative conditions associated with self-destructive behavior (i.e., family dysfunction, history of suicide attempt, etc.) can reduce the risk of suicide.

Community crisis hotlines also offer an opportunity for the secondary prevention of suicide. Hotlines can provide adolescents with immediate, confidential access to a person (usually a volunteer) who can offer emotional support and referral. The rationale supporting hotlines is that suicides are often associated with both an acute stressful event and with ambivalence about ending one's life (29). Some support for the effectiveness of these programs is supplied in a study by Miller, who found that the presence of a community prevention center hotline reduced the rate of suicide among young white females (60). In general, however, hotlines have not had a large impact, possibly because those at risk for suicide may not know of their existence (29, 59). A somewhat older study by Slem and Cotler (61), however, demonstrated that targeted advertising of a hotline service to high school students can effectively increase name recognition and utilization.

Treatment options for adolescent major depression disorder include psychotherapy, family therapy, cognitive-behavioral therapy, relaxation training, and antidepressant medication. Each modality has been shown to have some benefit in relieving depression, and multimodal approaches are usually warranted. Studies have failed to determine, however, a single most effective therapeutic intervention (11, 62–64).

Clinical Application

In light of the sizable number of adolescents who suffer fluctuations in depressive symptomatology, physicians must be careful to determine the persistence of mood changes and whether this has associated behavioral changes. Special attention should be given to a sudden decline in school grades and to social isolation. A more in-depth assessment of adolescents with these symptoms should be done to identify those who have a major depressive disorder.

The identification of suicidal risk is managed in one of two ways. Adolescents who express acute suicidal intent, including a plan for how they would act on their wish, are at high risk for self-destructive behavior. They should be kept safe from self-harm and have an immediate mental health evaluation. Adolescents who have cumulative risks for suicide—especially prior suicidal behavior, depression, and alcohol or other drug use—but who are not actively suicidal, must be assessed to determine the degree of their overall risk. In all cases of potential suicide, there must be an assessment of the availability of firearms and lethal medications in the home.

REFERENCES

1. Zill N, Schoenborn CA. Developmental, learning and emotional problems: Health of our nation's children, United States, 1988. Advance Data from Vital and Health Statistics, #190. Hyattsville, MD: National Center for Health Statistics, 1990.

2. Offer D, Ostrov E, Howard KI: Epidemiology of mental health and mental illness among adolescents. In: Call JD, Cohen RL, Harrison SI, Berlin IN, Stone LA, eds. Basic Handbook of Child Psychiatry. New York: Basic Books, 1987.

3. Regier DA, Boyd JH, Burke JD, et al. One-month prevalence of mental disorders in the United States. Arch Gen Psychiatry 1988;45:977–986.

4. Burke KC, Burke JD, Rae DS, Regier DA. Comparing age at onset of major depression and other psychiatric disorders by birth cohorts in five US communities. Arch Gen Psychiatry 1991; 48:789–795.

5. Burke KC, Burke JD, Regier DA, Rae DS. Age at onset of selected mental disorders in five community populations. Arch Gen Psychiatry 1990;47:511–518.

6. American School Health Association. The National Adolescent Student Health Survey: A Report on the Health of America's Youth. Kent, OH: American School Health Association, 1989.

7. Fleming JE, Offord DR. Epidemiology of childhood depressive disorders: a critical review. J Am Acad Child Adoles Psychiatry 1990;29:571–580.

8. Garrison CZ, Schluchter MD, Schoenback VJ, Kaplan BK. Epidemiology of depressive symptoms in young adolescents. J Am Acad Child Adoles Psychiatry 1989;28:343–351.

9. Whitaker A, Johnson J, Shaffer D, et al. Uncommon troubles in young people: prevalence estimates of selected psychiatric disorders in a nonreferred adolescent population. Arch Gen Psychiatry 1990;47:487–496.

10. Kandel D, Davies M. Epidemiology of depressive mood in adolescents: an empirical study. Arch Gen Psychiatry 1982;39:1205–1212.

11. Aylward GP. Understanding and treatment of childhood depression. J Pediatr 1985;107:1–9.

12. Weissman MM, Gammon GD, John K, et al. Children of depressed parents. Arch Gen Psychiatry 1987;44:847–853.

13. Crumley FE. Substance abuse and adolescent suicidal behavior. JAMA 1990;263:3051–3056.

14. Kaplan SL, Landa B, Weinhold C, Shenker IR. Adverse health behaviors and depressive symptomatology in adolescents. J Am Acad Child Adoles Psychiatry 1984;23:595–601.

15. Fleming JE, Boyle MH, Offord DR. The outcome of adolescent depression in the Ontario Child Health Study follow-up. J Am Acad Child Adoles Psychiatry 1993;32:28–33.

16. Kandel DB, Davies M. Adult sequelae of adolescent depressive symptoms. Arch Gen Psychiatry 1986;43:255–262.

17. Harrington R, Fudge H, Rutter M, Pickles A, Hill J. Adult outcomes of childhood and adolescent depression I: psychiatric status. Arch Gen Psychiatry 1990;47:465–473.

18. Centers for Disease Control. Attempted Suicide Among High School Students—United States, 1990. MMWR 1991;40:633–635.

19. Centers for Disease Control. Youth Suicide in the United States, 1970–1980. Washington, DC: Department of Health and Human Services, 1986.

20. Grossman DC, Milligan BC, Deyo RA. Risk factors for suicide attempts among Navajo adolescents. Am J Public Health 1991;81:870–874.

21. American Medical Association, Council on Scientific Affairs. Health status of detained and incarcerated youth. JAMA 1989;263:1939–1942.

22. Remafedi G, Farrow JA, Deisher RW. Risk factors for attempted suicide in gay and bisexual youth. Pediatrics 1991;87:869–875.

23. Schwartz AJ, Whitaker LC. Suicide among college students: assessment, treatment, and intervention. In: Blumenthal SJ, Kupfer DJ, eds. Suicide Over the Life Cycle: Risk Factors, Assessment, and Treatment of Suicidal Patients. Washington DC: American Psychiatric Press, 1990:303–340.

24. Garrison C, Jackson K, Addy C, McKeown R, Waller J. Suicidal behaviors in young adolescents. Am J Epidemiol 1991;10:1005–1014.

25. Joffe R, Offord D, Bolye M. Ontario Child Health Study: Suicidal behavior in youth age 12–16 years. Am J Psychiatry 1988;145:1420–1423.

26. Hawton K. Suicide and Attempted Suicide Among Children and Adolescents. Beverly Hills: Sage Publications, 1986:121–153.

27. McIntire MS, Angle CR, et al. Recurrent adolescent suicide behavior. Pediatrics 1977;60:605–608.

28. Angle CR, O'Brien TP, McIntire MS. Adolescent self-poisoning: a nine-year follow-up. Dev Behav Pediatr 1983;4:83–87.

29. Shaffer D, Garland A, Gould M, Fisher P, Trautman P. Preventing teenage suicide: a critical review. J Am Acad Child Adoles Psychiatry 1988;27:675–687.

30. Brent DA, Kalas R, Edelbrock C, Costello AJ, Dulcan MK, Conover N. Psychopathology and its relationship to suicidal ideation in childhood and adolescence. J Am Acad Child Psychiatry 1986;25:666–673.

31. Brent DA, Perper JA, Goldstein CE, et al. Risk factors for adolescent suicide: a comparison of adolescent suicide victims with suicidal inpatients. Arch Gen Psychiatry 1988;45:581–588.

32. Pfeffer CR, Newcorn J, Kaplan G, Mizruchi MS, Plutchik R. Suicidal behavior in adolescent psychiatric inpatients. Am Acad Child Adoles Psychiatry 1988;27:357–361.

33. Apter A, Bleich A, Plutchik R, Mendelsohn S, Tyano S. Suicidal behavior, depression, and conduct disorder in hospitalized adolescents. J Am Acad Child Adoles Psychiatry 1988;27:696–699.

34. Shafii M, Steltz-Lenarsky J, Derrick AM, Beckner C, Whittinghill JR. Comorbidity of mental disorders in the postmortem diagnosis of completed suicide in children and adolescents. J Affect Disord 1988;15:227–233.

35. Slap GB, Vorters DF, Chaudhuri S, Centor RM. Risk factors for attempted suicide during adolescence. Pediatrics 1989;84:762–772.

36. Swedo SE, Rettewi DC, Kuppenheimer M, Lum D, Dolan S, Goldberger E. Can adolescent suicide attempters be distinguished from at-risk adolescents? Pediatrics 1991;88:620–629.

37. Riggs S, Alario AJ, McHorney C. Health-risk behaviors and attempted suicide in adolescents who report prior maltreatment. J Pediatrics 1990;116:815–821.

38. Trautman PD, Shaffer D. Treatment of Child and Adolescent Suicide Attempters. In: Sudak H, Ford A, Rushforth N, eds. Suicide in the Young. Boston: John Wright, 1984:307–323.

39. Carlson CA, Cantwell DP. Suicidal behavior and depression in children and adolescents. J Am Acad Child Adoles Psychiatry 1982;21:361–368.

40. Gould M, Shaffer D. The impact of suicide in television movies: evidence of imitation. N Engl J Med 1986;315:690–694.

41. Brent DA, Perper JA, Allman CJ, Moritz GM, Wartella ME, Zelenak JP. The presence and accessibility of firearms in the homes of adolescent suicides: a case-control study. JAMA 1991;266:2989–2995.

42. Brent DA, Perper JA, Allman CJ. Alcohol, firearms, and suicide among youth: temporal trends in Allegheny County, Pennsylvania, 1960–1983. JAMA 1987;257:3369–3372.

43. Sloan JH, Rivara FP, Reay DT. Firearm regulations and rates of suicide: a comparison of two metropolitan areas. N Engl J Med 1990;322:369–373.

44. American Psychiatric Association. Diagnostic and Statistical Manual of Mental Disorders (3rd edition revised). Washington, DC: American Psychiatric Association, 1987.

45. Roberts RE, Lewinsohn PM, Seeley JR. Screening for adolescent depression: a comparison of depression scales. J Am Acad Child Adoles Psychiatry 1991;30:58–66.

46. Schubiner H, Robin A. Screening adolescents for depression and parent-teenager conflict in an ambulatory medical setting: a preliminary investigation. Pediatrics 1990;85:813–818.

47. Coulehan JL, Schulberg HC, Block MR. The efficiency of depression questionnaires for case finding in primary medical care. J Gen Intern Med 1989;4:541–547.

48. US Preventive Services Task Force: Guide to Clinical Preventive Services: An Assessment of the Effectiveness of 169 Interventions. Baltimore: Williams & Wilkins, 1989:265–269.

49. Lewinsohn PM, Rohde P, Seeley JR. Psychosocial characteristics of adolescents with a history of suicide attempt. J Am Acad Child Adoles Psychiatry 1993;32:60–68.

50. Garrison CZ, McKeown RE, Valois RF, Vincent ML. Aggression, substance use, and suicidal behaviors in high school students. Am J Public Health 1993;83:179–184.

51. Brown LK, Overholser J, Spirito A, Fritz GK. The correlates of planning in adolescent suicide attempts. J Am Acad Child Adoles Psychiatry 1991;30:95–99.

52. Goldberg ID, Roghmann KJ, McInerny TK, Burke JD. Mental health problems among children seen in pediatric practice: prevalence and management. Pediatrics 1984;73:278–293.

53. Schor EL. Use of health care services by children and diagnoses received during presumably stressful life transitions. Pediatrics 1986;77:834–841.

54. Starfield B, Gross E, Wood M, et al. Psychosocial and psychosomatic diagnoses in primary care of children. Pediatrics 1980;66:159–167.

55. Hodgman CH, Roberts FN. Adolescent suicide and the pediatrician. J Pediatrics 1982;101:118–123.

56. Costello EJ, Edelbrock C, Costello AJ, Dulcan MK, Burns BJ, Brent D. Psychopathology in pediatric primary care: the new hidden morbidity. Pediatrics 1988;82:415–424.

57. Slap GB, Vorters DF, Khalid N, Margulies SR, Forke CM. Adolescent suicide attempters: do physicians recognize them? J Adolesc Health 1992;13:286–292.

58. Chang G, Warner V, Weissman MM. Physicians' recognition of psychiatric disorders in children and adolescents. Am J Dis Child 1988;142:736–739.

59. Eddy DM, Wolpert RL, Rosenberg ML. Estimating the effectiveness of interventions to prevent youth suicides: a report to the Secretary's Task Force on Youth Suicide. In: Report of the Secretary's Task Force on Youth Suicide (Vol 4). Strategies for the Prevention of Youth Suicide. Washington, DC: Alcohol, Drug Abuse, and Mental Health Administration. DHHS Publication No. (ADM) 89–1624, 1989:37–45.

60. Miller HL, Coombs DW, Leeper JD, Barton SN. An analysis of the effects of suicide prevention facilities on suicide rates in the United States. Am J Public Health 1984;74:340–343.

61. Slem CM, Cotler S. Crisis phone services: evaluation of a hotline program. Am J Community Psychol 1973;1:219–227.

62. Reynolds WM, Coats KI. A comparison of cognitive-behavioral therapy and relaxation training for the treatment of depression in adolescents. J Counsel Clin Psychol 1986;54:653–660.

63. Ryan ND, Puig-Antick J, Cooper T, et al. Imipramine in adolescent major depression: plasma level and clinical response. Acta Psychiatr Scand 1986;73:275–288.

64. Keller MB, Lavori PW, Beardslee WR, Wunder J, Ryan N. Depression in children and adolescents: new data on "undertreatment" and a literature review on the efficacy of available treatments. J Affect Disord 1991;21:163–171.

CHAPTER 13

Rationale and Recommendation: Emotional, Physical, and Sexual Abuse

PREVENTION STRATEGY

GAPS recommends that during the annual preventive service visit physicians screen adolescents for emotional, physical, or sexual abuse. If abuse is suspected, additional evaluation will be needed to determine the circumstances surrounding the abuse: physicians should note the presence of physical signs of abuse (i.e., signs of burns or scars); and the degree of emotional, physical, or psychosocial sequelae (i.e., suicide ideation, involvement in health-risk behaviors, such as alcohol and other drug use or unsafe sexual practices, etc.). Adolescents who are suffering sequelae of the abuse need mental health counseling and should be referred for evaluation and treatment. In all states, abuse is an offense that must be reported to the appropriate child protective authorities. Since reporting of abuse breaches confidentiality, physicians must ensure that their adolescent patients are counseled on the procedures and actions that will follow disclosure. Physician guidelines for screening for abuse are addressed in GAPS Recommendation 21.

DISCUSSION

Adolescent maltreatment includes physical abuse, emotional abuse, sexual abuse, and neglect. The following definitions are used in GAPS:

Physical abuse ". . . implies injury of a non-accidental nature with a significant risk of death, disfigurement, and/or prolonged disability" (1). In contrast to assault, ". . . the injury must have been inflicted by the parent, caretaker, or legal guardian."

"*Neglect* implies the failure of the caretaker to minimally provide adequate food, shelter, clothing, education, and health care" (1).

Emotional abuse ". . . may include acts of omission, such as rejection or lack of discipline, or commission, such as degrading comments or public humiliation" (1).

Sexual abuse can be defined as ". . . the involvement of dependent, developmentally immature children and adolescents in sexual activities that they do not understand, to which they are unable to give informed consent, or that are inappropriate for family roles" (2). GAPS makes the distinction between sexual abuse, which is perpetrated by a relative, and sexual assault (i.e., molestation, rape, etc.) in which the offender is a stranger or an acquaintance. Sexual assault is discussed in Chapter 7.

The rate of reported cases of maltreatment in 12–14-year-old adolescents has increased from 12 cases per 1,000 in 1980 to 23 cases per 1,000 in 1986 (3, 4). Reported rates for adolescents age 15–17 increased from 14 cases per 1,000 in 1980 to 23 cases per 1,000 in 1986 (the 1986 rate of 23 cases per 1,000 is the corrected calculation from the rate originally published) (5). When analyzed by type of abuse, the reported rate of physical abuse doubled during this period, while the reported rate of sexual abuse tripled (4). Although reported abuse has increased since the late 1970s, it is not clear if this change represents an actual increase in the amount of actual abuse or if it is the result of better reporting. In a meta-analysis comparing data obtained in the 1940s with data from studies done in the 1970s and 1980s, Feldman and associates estimated that sexual abuse has not actually increased (6). They concluded that increases in reporting probably resulted from passage of legislation mandating notification of abuse and changes in social climate toward increased child protection.

In 1990, state agencies received 1.7 million reports of abuse affecting approximately 2.7 million children (7). Adolescents are over-represented among these cases. For example, in a 1980 national incidence study, adolescents accounted for 47% of reported cases of child abuse and 42% of substantiated cases, although they represented only 38% of the total population under age 18 (3). Furthermore, in Minnesota investigators found that 42% of cases of maltreatment involved adolescents (8), while other investigators found that 31% of neglect reports, 42% of sexual abuse reports, and 19% of physical abuse reports in New York State involved adolescents (9). Maltreatment is more common among adolescent females than among adolescent males (3, 4). This gender difference is greatest for sexual abuse. Because abuse to males is often not reported unless there is severe injury, however, gender differences might not be as great as survey results suggest. Certain groups of adolescents, such as those who are mentally retarded, are especially vulnerable to maltreatment (10, 11).

Compared to younger children, abused adolescents are less likely to be reported to child protection agencies, and the abuse is less likely to be substantiated (4, 5, 12–15). The problem of under reporting is compounded when epidemiological studies of abuse rely only on cases reported by child protection agencies. Reasons for not reporting adolescent maltreatment include: (1) child protection agencies generally focus services on younger children and refer maltreated adolescents elsewhere for treatment; (2) due to low substantiation rates, adolescent victims less frequently qualify for service benefits than do younger children; and (3) abuse may be identified by a variety of service entry points (e.g., the justice system, mental health system, or alternative youth service system); abuse is just one of the many behaviors or problems on which these service entry points tend to focus.

The problem of under-reporting of adolescent maltreatment is emphasized by the results of a national survey in which only 39% of suspected adolescent abuse cases were reported to a child protection agency, compared to 76% of cases involving younger children (16). Even when reported to a child protection agency, however, adolescent maltreatment is less likely to be substantiated than is maltreatment of younger children, for several reasons (12–14).

First, adolescents experience less severe physical injuries than do younger children, thus reducing the likelihood that the abuse will be substantiated. Also, adolescents may be perceived as responsible for the abuse they experience because of misbehavior preceding the parental abuse or, in some cases, because they respond to abuse with an assault against the parent.

A distinction can be made between adolescent maltreatment that begins during childhood and continues, and maltreatment that begins during adolescence (16–19). Adolescent-onset abuse appears related to the inability of parents to adjust their disciplinary patterns to meet the characteristics of the child, and it occurs at periods of high family stress (16). In some cases, for example, abuse that occurs during early childhood ceases as parents and child develop more compatible disciplinary patterns, but it re-emerges during adolescence when parental authority is again challenged (18).

The arrival of adolescence causes a fundamental readjustment in family dynamics and communication patterns that is stressful for some families (20). The need of the adolescent for greater independence necessitates changes in parental behavior. Parents who have difficulty making these adjustments may resort to coercion and force. Although research data are sparse, families experiencing childhood-onset abuse are more likely to have multiple problems, intergenerational abuse, spousal abuse, and lower levels of income and education than are families with adolescent-onset abuse (12, 19). Due to its chronic nature, childhood-onset abuse may also have more serious and long-lasting effects on the victim. Parents who begin abuse during adolescence have been reported to be more amenable to treatment than those for whom abuse has been an established pattern since the youth's childhood (19).

The health consequences of adolescent abuse are gaining increased recognition. For example, adolescents who were sexually abused as younger children are more likely than other adolescents to have a major mood disorder; to attempt suicide; and to engage in premature sexual activity, substance and alcohol abuse, and delinquency (21–27). Sexually abused females are also at risk for emotional and sexual abuse problems as adults (28).

Abuse is a major factor leading adolescents to run away from home (29–31). For example, 28% of youths in one study who were seen in a shelter program reported that they had been abused, and more than two-thirds of these reported being abused more than five times (30). Another study reported that 38% of males and 73% of females who ran away from home did so to avoid further sexual abuse (31).

The association between maltreatment and involvement in health-risk behaviors is found for males as well as for females. Several of these behaviors, such as prostitution and intravenous drug abuse, place abused adolescents at risk for HIV infection (23). For example, in a study of 186 sexually active subjects, Zierler and associates found that survivors of prior sexual abuse were four times more likely than other young adults to report having worked as a prostitute (32). This association was independent of gender and IV drug abuse. A recent meta-analysis by Kendall-Tackett and associates synthesized information regarding the impact of sexual abuse on children (33). Symptoms of sexual abuse appeared to follow a developmental trajectory, where adolescents displayed a different group of symptoms than did younger children. For adolescents, the predominant constellation of symptoms included substance abuse (53%), depression (46%), withdrawn mood (45%), suicidal ideation (41%), and somatic complaints (34%). Overall, most children (50–66%) became less symptomatic with time, while some children (10–24%) worsened. Children who were older at assessment of the abusive incident appeared to have more symptoms than did those who were younger. Data were insufficient to draw conclusions regarding differences in symptomatology by age at onset of abuse.

Although most abused adolescents do not engage in violent behavior themselves, a prior history of abuse is a risk factor for later violent behavior

(34, 35). Rivera and Widom compared the rate of violent offenses among a group of 908 abused or neglected adults with a control group of 667 adults (36). Most of the sample were age 20–30. Although no group differences were found for violence committed as a juvenile, males and blacks who had been abused were significantly more likely to be arrested for violent offenses as adults.

JUSTIFICATION

The recommendation for screening for abuse is justified predominantly by strong national consensus, based on expert opinion, that early identification of abuse is necessary to protect the physical and emotional well-being of the adolescent.

What Is the Most Effective Way to Identify Adolescents Who Have Been Abused?

The diagnosis of maltreatment is made through a clinical interview, with corroborative evidence provided by findings from the physical examination. Inclusion of questions about abuse in the routine screening of adolescent patients has been shown to reveal previously undiagnosed cases of maltreatment, especially among males (37, 38). The behavioral and emotional signs of adolescent maltreatment are often ambiguous and easy to confuse with health problems presumed to result from normal development and behavior. Adolescent maltreatment can be "masked" by psychosomatic, emotional, or behavioral problems (39). Disclosure of abuse can occur accidentally, when abuse is discovered by chance, or by deliberate effort to tell someone of the incident (38).

In a study of 116 sexually abused children and adolescents, Sorenson and Snow found that most (74%) disclosures were accidental (38). These percentages changed sharply with age, however, so that among adolescents only 40% of disclosures were accidental. Sorenson and Snow concluded that disclosure was best described as a process, not an event. Most children do not reveal sexual abuse at the time of the initial interview, but rather go through stages including denial, tentative agreement to disclose, and then active disclosure. Recanting of an accusation is also common.

Identifying adolescents who have a history of abuse can serve to protect them from additional emotional and physical trauma. This is also the time to initiate the treatment process. Research on the effectiveness of treatment in improving the overall adjustment of adolescents has primarily focused on sexual abuse victims. Approaches used in child sexual abuse treatment programs include: (1) lay or paraprofessional approaches utilizing peer counseling and support groups, (2) group approaches using group therapy and education, (3) approaches relying primarily on individual counseling and case management, and (4) cognitive-behavioral therapy addressing abuse as a posttraumatic stress disorder. Surveys of treatment programs indicate that most clinicians prefer comprehensive, interdisciplinary family system treatments that combine elements of multiple approaches (40). Outcome studies, however, have tended to focus on categorical treatments employing a particular approach.

Evidence exists that group approaches are effective in improving adolescent adjustment as measured through psychological checklists, ability to discuss abuse, improved school performance, increased involvement in peer activities, and reduced revictimization and recanting (40). In children, cognitive-behavioral therapy, which includes components for parents, appears to significantly reduce self-reported depression, state and trait anxiety, avoidance behavior, and externalizing and internalizing of problems. The level of family functioning and family involvement in treatment are frequently cited as factors influencing the effectiveness of treatment (41, 42).

CLINICAL APPLICATION

Because of the sensitive nature of the issue, inquiries about abuse should be asked while physicians are alone with their adolescent patients. Maltreatment should be suspected when adolescents have unexplained bruises or fractures; vague, lower abdominal symptoms unrelated to obvious physical disease; involvement at an early age in health-risk behaviors, such as use of alcohol or other drugs and unsafe sexual behaviors; depression; failing academic performance; or unintended pregnancy or STD infections during early adolescence (e.g., prior to age 14). Emotional abuse and neglect are especially difficult to document and require that a link be determined between the presumed maltreatment and a negative health or emotional outcome.

Once a history of maltreatment is suspected or proven, the provider has a legal responsibility to report the case to the appropriate child protection agency. Although abuse is usually a reportable event, physicians must prepare the adolescent before disclosing the information to local authorities. The more acute the nature of the problem, the more quickly the report must be made. Because of the high rate of subsequent involvement in problem behavior, GAPS recommends that the primary provider continue to follow these adolescents and monitor their health.

As a primary prevention strategy, physicians are asked to provide health guidance to parents to help them adjust their parenting to meet the changing needs of their adolescents (see Chapter 2). During these sessions, family difficulties related to discipline can be identified and suggestions provided for improving parenting techniques.

REFERENCES

1. Richardson AC. Physical and Emotional Abuse. In: McAnarney ER, Kreipe R, Orr R, Comerci G, eds. Textbook of Adolescent Medicine. Philadelphia: WB Saunders Co, 1992:1119–1122.

2. Hibbard RA. Sexual Abuse. In: McAnarney ER, Kreipe R, Orr R, Comerci G, eds. Textbook of Adolescent Medicine. Philadelphia: WB Saunders Co, 1992:1123–1127.

3. US Department of Health and Human Services. National Study of the Incidence and Severity of Child Abuse and Neglect: 1981. Washington, DC: US Government Printing Office, 1981.

4. US Department of Health and Human Services. National Study of the Incidence and Severity of Child Abuse and Neglect: 1988. Washington, DC: US Government Printing Office, 1988.

5. American Medical Association, Council on Scientific Affairs. Adolescents as victims of family violence. Chicago: American Medical Association, 1992.

6. Feldman W, Feldman E, Goodman JT, McGrath PJ, et al. Is childhood sexual abuse really increasing in prevalence? An analysis of the evidence. Pediatrics 1991;88:29–33.

7. National Center for Child Abuse and Neglect. National Child Abuse and Neglect Data System Working Paper 1, 1990 Summary Data Component. Washington, DC: USDHHS Publication No. (ACF) 92–30361, 1992.

8. Blum R, Runyan C. Adolescent abuse: the dimensions of the problem. J Adolesc Health Care 1980;1:121–126.

9. Powers JL, Eckenrode J. The maltreatment of adolescents. Child Abuse Negl 1988;12:189–199.

10. Chamberlain A, Rauh J, Passer A, McGrath M, Burket R. Issues in fertility control for mentally retarded female adolescents: I. Sexual activity, sexual abuse, and contraception. Pediatrics 1984;73:445–450.

11. Tharinger D, Horton CB, Millea S. Sexual abuse and exploitation of children and adults with mental retardation and other handicaps. Child Abuse Negl 1990;14:301–312.

12. Berdie J, Berdie M, Wexler S, Fisher B. An Empirical Study of Families Involved in Adolescent Maltreatment: Final Report. Grant No. 90-CA-837101. Washington, DC: National Center on Child Abuse and Neglect, USDHHS, 1983.

13. Miller A. Thou Shall Not Be Aware: Society's Betrayal of the Child. New York: Farrar, Straus & Giroux, 1984.

14. Doueck JJ, Hideki AI, Love SS, Gilchrist L. Adolescent maltreatment: themes from the empirical literature. J Interper Violence 1987;2:139–153.

15. Fisher B, Berdie J. Adolescent abuse and neglect: issues of incidence, intervention, and service delivery. Child Abuse Negl 1978;2:173–192.

16. Fisher B, Berdie J, Cook J, Day N. Adolescent Abuse and Neglect: Intervention Strategies. Washington, DC: USDHHS Publication No. 80–30266, 1980.

17. Lourie IS. Family dynamics and the abuse of adolescents: a case for a developmental phase-specific model of child abuse. Child Abuse Negl 1979;3:967–974.

18. Libby P, Bybee R. The physical abuse of adolescents. J Soc Issues 1979;35:101–126.

19. Garbarino J, Schellenbach C, Sebes J, et al. Troubled Youth, Troubled Families: Understanding Families At-Risk for Adolescent Maltreatment. New York: Aldine de Gruyter Publishing Co, 1986.

20. Hill JP, Holmbeck GN, Marlow L, Green TM, Lynch ME. Pubertal status and parent-child relations in families of seventh-grade boys. J Early Adolesc 1985;5:31–44.

21. Polit DF, White CM, Morton TD. Child sexual abuse and premarital intercourse among high-risk adolescents. J Adolesc Health Care 1990;11:231–234.

22. Vermund SH, Alexander-Rodriguez T, Macleod S, Kelly KF. History of sexual abuse in incarcerated adolescents with gonorrhea or syphilis. J Adolesc Health Care 1990;11:449–452.

23. Riggs S, Alario AJ, McHorney C. Health-risk behaviors and attempted suicide in adolescents who report prior maltreatment. J Pediatr 1990;116:815–821.

24. Browne A, Finkelhor D. Impact of child sexual abuse: a review of the research. Psychol Bull 1986;99:66–77.

25. Dembo R, Dertke M, Borders S. The relationship between physical and sexual abuse and tobacco, alcohol, and illicit drug use among youths in a juvenile detention center. Inter J Addict 1988;23:351–378.

26. Hibbard RA, Brack CJ, Rauch S, Orr DP. Abuse, feelings, and health behaviors in a student population. Am J Dis Child 1988;142:326–330.

27. Hibbard RA, Ingersoll GM, Orr DP. Behavioral risk, emotional risk, and child abuse among adolescents in a nonclinical setting. Pediatrics 1990;86:896–901.

28. Bachmann GA, Moeller TP, Benett J. Childhood sexual abuse and the consequences in adult women. Obstet Gynecol 1988;71:631–642.

29. American Medical Association, Council on Scientific Affairs. Health care needs of homeless and runaway youths. JAMA 1989;262:1358–1361.

30. Kurtz PD, Kurtz GL, Jarvis SV. Problems of maltreated runaway youth. Adolescence 1991;26:543–555.

31. McCormack A, Janus MD, Burges AW. Runaway youths and sexual victimization: gender differences in adolescent runaway population. Child Abuse Negl 1986;10:387–395.

32. Zierler S, Feingold L, Laufer D, Velentgas P, Kantrowitz-Gordon R, Mayer K. Adult survivors of childhood sexual abuse and subsequent risk of HIV infection. Am J Public Health 1991;81:572–575.

33. Kendall-Tackett KA, Williams LM, Finkelhor D. Impact of sexual abuse on children: a review and synthesis of recent empirical studies. Psychol Bull 1993;113:164–180.

34. Widom CS. Child abuse, neglect, and adult behavior: research design and findings on criminality, violence, and child abuse. Am J Orthopsychiatry 1989;59:355–367.

35. Widom CS. Does violence beget violence? A critical examination of the literature. Psychol Bull 1989;106:3–28.

36. Rivera B, Widom CS. Childhood victimization and violent offending. Violence Vict 1990;5:19–35.

37. Johnson RL, Shrier DK. Sexual victimization of boys: experience at an adolescent medicine clinic. J Adolesc Health Care 1985;6:372–376.

38. Sorenson T, Snow B. How children tell: the process of disclosure in child sexual abuse. Child Welfare 1991;70:3–15.

39. Hunter RS, Kilstrom N, Loda F. Sexually abused children: identifying masked presentations in a medical setting. Child Abuse Negl 1985;9:17–25.

40. Kitchur M, Bell R. Group psychotherapy with preadolescent sexual abuse victims: literature review and description of an inner-city group. Int J Group Psychother 1989;39:285–310.

41. Deblinger E, McLeer SV, Henry D. Cognitive-behavioral treatment for sexually abused children suffering from posttraumatic stress: preliminary findings. J Am Acad Child Adoles Psychiatry 1990;29:747–752.

42. Pfeiffer SI, Strzelecki SC. Inpatient psychiatric treatment of children and adolescents: a review of outcome studies. J Am Acad Child Adoles Psychiatry 1990;29:847–853.

CHAPTER 14

Rationale and Recommendation: Primary Learning Disorders

PREVENTION STRATEGY

GAPS recommends that all adolescents be screened annually for academic and behavioral problems related to school. These problems are often an early sign of learning disorders and can have serious health consequences. Adolescents who have repeated truancy or poor or declining school grades should have a thorough physical, behavioral, and emotional evaluation as well as an assessment of academic ability and family environment. Information from teachers and records of scholastic aptitude testing are essential. The evaluation and management should be coordinated with school personnel. Conditions that can interfere with school performance include a specific learning disability (LD), attention deficit hyperactivity disorder (ADHD), medical problems (e.g., hearing or vision deficiency), depression, conduct disorder, and substance abuse. Screening for hearing and vision are usually performed within the schools and are not, therefore, addressed by GAPS. Screening for conduct disorder is not included in GAPS because adolescents with this condition usually have prominent behavioral symptoms. Guidelines for screening for substance use and for depression are addressed in GAPS Recommendations 15 and 20, respectively. Physician guidelines for screening adolescents for learning disorders are addressed in GAPS Recommendation 22.

DISCUSSION

As described in various national reports, there is a growing realization of the important connection between learning and health (1, 2). Health is a necessary prerequisite to learning, which in turn helps fosters emotional well-being and developmental adjustment. Although school performance can also be affected by social and cultural factors, physical handicaps, depression and other emotional disorders, and mental retardation, this GAPS recommendation only addresses screening for primary learning disorders and not other conditions that can interfere with learning.

In the context of GAPS, a primary learning disorder refers to a central nervous system condition that results from a genetic or biological cause that places an adolescent at risk for not performing academic tasks at normative levels for age. This definition includes both LD, including various types of developmental dysfunctions and ADHD, with or without hyperactivity. Youth with LD manifest a discrepancy between intellectual ability and academic achievement due to a deficit in one or more psychological processes such as attention, memory, or perception (3–5). Specific learning disabilities should be suspected in adolescents who have a chronic history of academic difficulty in selected classes (e.g., math and reading). Grades in classes that do not rely heavily on the deficient skill may be satisfactory. Early treatment is necessary to help these adolescents with remedial training and to prevent them from falling further behind academically. Even with treatment, however, LD during childhood may adversely affect later educational and social achievement (5). GAPS will place greater emphasis on ADHD than on LD because of the larger role primary care physicians have in the identification and management of this disorder.

The hallmark symptoms of ADHD include a developmentally inappropriate low level of sustained attention, diminished impulse control, and excessive physical activity. Results of longitudinal studies suggest that children with ADHD will follow one of three trajectories during adolescence: (1) they will outgrow their symptoms; (2) symptoms will persist, but in a modified form that causes only mild difficulties; or (3) symptoms will persist, but will become associated with severe behavioral and emotional disorders (6). It is this later group of adolescents that presents the greatest health concerns. As many as 40% of children with ADHD will have a co-diagnosis of conduct disorder and engage in delinquent activities and other problem behaviors (7). From 20–50% of children with ADHD, however, are generally symptom-free during adolescence, while the remainder will continue during adolescence to exhibit symptoms of overactivity, impulsivity, and/or short attention span (7–10).

During adolescence, the associated problems of low self-esteem and disruptive behavior may become dominant features and overshadow the impulsivity, poor peer relationships, and academic difficulties that characterized the preadolescent (11, 12). Adolescents with ADHD are more likely than their peers to repeat a school grade, exhibit behavioral problems in school, and attend special education classes (7–10, 13). The long-term negative effects of ADHD may be somewhat overstated. Care must be taken when interpreting studies on ADHD because poor outcomes appear related to the presence of conduct disorder in addition to the consequences of hyperactivity, impulsivity, and inattention. With the recent emphasis on the identification and management of ADHD in the primary care setting, many children with ADHD are not being referred for additional psychiatric evaluation and treatment. Follow-up studies of non-referred adolescents are needed to determine the long-term consequences for less disturbed adolescents who do not have conduct disorder.

Although both LD and ADHD are present at early ages, the conditions are not usually identified until the child starts school. Some youths may have performed well enough academically to pass undiagnosed through elementary school or even junior high. Moving into secondary school, however, adolescents experience an increased complexity of academic material and evolving peer pressures to engage in social rather than academic pursuits (14). These changes may be more problematic than the academically marginal adolescent with a learning disability can manage, and they may lead to declining school performance. Results from the National Health Interview Survey of Child Health support the notion that many children with a learning disorder go through early school years without being identified.

Using data from the National Health Interview Survey, Zill and Schoenborn found that the proportion of children reported by parents to have a learning problem increased from 1.6% at age 3–5, to 6.8% at age 6–11, and to 8.8% at age 12–17 (3). For 16% of children, their problem was not detected until late elementary or secondary school. Results from other studies confirm that an estimated 3–7% of children and adolescents have a specific learning disability, while approximately 5–6% have ADHD (4, 15–18). Although LD and ADHD are different conditions, there is substantial overlap. Approximately 10–30% of youths with one disorder will have the other disorder as well (4, 19–21). Learning disorders are much more common in males than in females by a rate of over 2-to-1; somewhat more common in whites than in blacks; and somewhat more in non-Hispanics than in Hispanics (3). These rate comparisons come from parent reports and must be interpreted with caution. There is some indication that rates of learning problems determined either by adolescents referred to mental health clinics or by teacher and parents are biased because males tend to have more associated behavioral manifestations and, therefore, are more readily identified than females (16).

Justification

Justification for the GAPS recommendation to screen adolescents for learning disorders is based on a large burden of suffering, the well-delineated criteria for identifying adolescents with ADHD, and the effectiveness of treatment.

How Are Adolescents with a Learning Disorder Best Identified?

A learning disorder should be suspected among adolescents who have chronically low or declining school grades, repeated truancies, and behavioral difficulties. Manifestations of ADHD usually appear in varying degrees of severity in school, at home, and in other social situations. Symptoms increase under stress and when sustained attention is necessary. The symptoms of inattention, impulsivity, and hyperactivity are manifested by not completing requested tasks, difficulty organizing work, interrupting when others are speaking, impatience with peers, excessive fidgeting when seated, and an inability to regulate behavior (22). During adolescence, these symptoms may become more subtle and overshadowed by associated problem behaviors. Although problems with conduct might be prominent, care should be taken to ensure that adolescents who engage in delinquent activity or in problem behaviors do not also have a learning disorder.

A diagnosis of ADHD requires a multidimensional assessment of: the adolescent's past academic, behavioral, and medical history; emotional status; family and environmental influences; and cognitive abilities (23). In addition to the clinical interview, information should be also be obtained from parents and the school. Assessment questionnaires, such as those developed by Conners, have been created to help standardize behavioral observations by both parents and teachers (24, 25). These questionnaires have proven highly robust in identifying adolescents with ADHD (26) and can be administrated and evaluated by primary care physicians. Referral for psychoeducational testing is also necessary to determine cognitive abilities and to determine if there is a coexisting diagnosis of LD. Psychoeducational testing should be done by professionals trained in administrating these procedures and evaluating the results. Psychiatric criteria necessary for a diagnosis of ADHD are presented in Table 14.1

The diagnosis of ADHD can only be made in the absence of other medical or emotional conditions that could cause a similar constellation of symptoms. Basic medical conditions (such as poor vision and hearing) and mental conditions (such as recurrent or severe depression, mental retardation, or substance abuse) should also be considered when evaluating the adolescent experiencing academic failure.

Table 14.1. Diagnostic Criteria for Attention Deficit Hyperactivity Disorder

Symptoms must have lasted at least six months with onset before the age of seven. To make a diagnosis of ADHD, adolescents must have at least eight of the following:

1. Often fidgets when seated, or reports feelings of restlessness

2. Has difficulty remaining seated when required to do so

3. Is easily distracted by extraneous stimuli

4. Has difficulty awaiting turn in games or group situations

5. Often bursts out answers before questions have been completed

6. Has difficulty following through on instructions from others (not due to oppositional behavior or failure of comprehension)

7. Has difficulty sustaining attention in tasks or play activities

8. Often shifts from one uncompleted activity to another

9. Has difficulty playing quietly

10. Often talks excessively

11. Often interrupts or intrudes on others

12. Often does not seem to listen to what is being said

13. Often loses things necessary for tasks or activities

14. Often engages in physically dangerous activities without considering possible consequences

Source: Diagnostic and Statistical Manual of Mental Disorders (3rd edition revised). Washington, DC American Psychiatric Association, 1987.

Are Interventions for ADHD Effective?

Various modalities have been used in the treatment of ADHD. These include stimulant medication, behavioral modification for both school and home, psychotherapy, family therapy, and cognitive counseling to help adolescents develop more appropriate problem-solving strategies (13, 27). Although research on multimodal interventions has been scarce, this approach appears to enhance treatment intensity and establish a framework for more promising outcomes. Stimulant medication, as an isolated intervention, remains the most widely used therapy for ADHD (18). In one study, Wolraich and associates found that over 70% of physicians prescribed stimulant medications for adolescents 10–13 years old with ADHD (18). Behavioral modification was used as a treatment for ADHD by 50–70% of physicians. Data from this study also exposed the mistaken belief that physicians were more hesitant to prescribe stimulant medication for older (over 14) compared to younger adolescents (under 15), and that some physicians still prescribed special diets and megavitamins for the treatment of ADHD.

Although there is considerable controversy regarding the effect of medication on long-term academic achievement and social development, stimulants do appear to have at least a short-term beneficial effect. For example, McBride conducted a double-blind crossover study to assess the effect of treatment with methylphenidate in 73 ADHD children between the age of 6 and 17 (28). Sixty-nine percent of the subjects improved while on the medication; the majority of these had sustained improvement in their symptoms for at least one year. The results of other studies also support the concept that approximately half of adolescents with ADHD show a favorable response to stimulant medication (11). Studies comparing the effect of stimulant medication, such as methylphenidate (Ritalin), dextroamphetamine (Dexedrine), and pemoline (Cylert) with placebo also verify that drug therapy is effective in reducing the immediate symptoms of impulsivity and increasing attention span (13, 28–30).

Benefits from stimulant medications, however, are not consistently associated with long-term improvement in school grades, problem behavior, or social measures (13, 29, 30). One reason for this is that follow-up study samples often include subjects with both ADHD and conduct disorder. Although both disorders share similar symptoms and a dual diagnosis is common, the majority of adolescents with ADHD do not have a conduct disorder (7, 9). Conduct disorder has a more guarded prognosis and is not usually responsive to treatment with stimulant medication. Other reasons for the lack of a long-term effect from stimulant medication include the possibility that drug treatment alone is not a sufficient intervention, that the medications are not prescribed long enough during adolescence, and that there is a failure to adhere to the treatment recommendations.

Side effects from medications are relatively common and include loss of appetite, weight loss, insomnia, headaches, dry mouth, and shakiness (29). These side effects are usually transient, however, and reverse when medications are stopped or decreased. There are no behavioral, social, or biochemical markers that indicate which adolescents with ADHD will benefit most from medications (28, 30).

CLINICAL APPLICATION

Because of the central role that educational achievement has in the life of adolescents, academic performance is one of the more sensitive and objective markers used to assess psychosocial adjustment and development. Adolescents who are identified as performing poorly in school should be assessed to determine causes for this problem. The causes include physical conditions, emotional disorders, and substance abuse disorders, as well as learning disorders. The evaluation for LD and ADHD will necessitate interviewing adolescents and their parents, obtaining and reviewing academic records from the school, and referral for psychoeducational testing. In many school districts, testing can be provided by the school psychologist. A management plan that includes counseling and special educational assistance, in addition to behavioral and, possibly, stimulant medication, should be developed and coordinated with the school.

REFERENCES

1. National Commission on the Role of the School and the Community in Improving Adolescent Health. Code Blue: Uniting for Healthier Youth. Chicago: American Medical Association, 1990.
2. Carnegie Council on Adolescent Development. Turning Points. Washington, DC: Carnegie Council on Adolescent Development, Carnegie Corporation of New York, 1989.
3. Zill N, Schoenborn CA. Developmental, Learning and Emotional Problems: Health of Our Nation's Children, United States, 1988. Advance Data from Vital and Health Statistics, #190. Hyattsville, MD: National Center for Health Statistics, 1990.
4. Silver LB. Controversial approaches to treating learning disabilities and attention deficit disorder. Am J Dis Child 1986;140:1045–1052.

5. Hartzell HE, Compton C. Learning disability: 10-year follow-up. Pediatrics 1984;74:1058–1064.

6. Cantwell DP. Pharmacotherapy of ADD in adolescents: what do we know, where should we go, how should we do it? Psychopharm Bull 1985;21:251–257.

7. Barkely RA, Fischer M, Edelbrock CS, Smallish L. The adolescent outcome of hyperactive children diagnosed by research criteria: I. An 8-year prospective follow-up study. J Am Acad Child Adoles Psychiatry 1990;29:546–557.

8. Satterfield JH, Hoppe CM, Schell AM. A prospective study of delinquency in 110 adolescent boys with attention deficit disorder and 88 normal adolescent boys. Am J Psychiatry 1982;139:795–798.

9. Weiss G, Hechtman L, Perlman T. Hyperactives as young adults: school, employer, and self-rating scales obtained during ten-year follow-up evaluation. Am J Orthopsychiatry 1978;48:438–445.

10. Gittleman R, Mannuzza S, Shenker R, Bonagura N: Hyperactive boys almost grown up. Arch Gen Psychiatry 1985;42:937–947.

11. Brown RT, Borden KA. Hyperactivity at adolescence. Some misconceptions and new directions. J Clin Child Psychol 1986;15:194–209.

12. Brown RT, Borden KA, Wynne ME, Spunt AL, Clingerman ST. Compliance with pharmacological and cognitive treatment for attention deficit disorder. J Am Acad Child Adoles Psychiatry 1987;26:521–526.

13. Hechtman L. Adolescent outcome of hyperactive children treated with stimulants in childhood: a review. Psychopharm Bull 1985;21:178–191.

14. Simmons RG. Social context and adolescent development. Paper presented at the Health Futures of Adolescence Conference, Daytona Beach, FL, April 1986.

15. McGee R, Feehan M, Williams S, Partridge F, Silva PA, Kelly J. DSM-III disorders in a large sample of adolescents. J Am Acad Child Adoles Psychiatry 1990;29:611–619.

16. Shaywitz SE, Shaywitz BA, Fletcher JM, Escobar MD. Prevalence of reading disability in boys and girls: results of the Connecticut Longitudinal Study. JAMA 1990;264:998–1002.

17. Szatmari P, Offord DR, Boyle MH. Ontario Child Health Study: prevalence of attention deficit disorder with hyperactivity. J Child Psychol Psychiatry 1989;30:219–230.

18. Wolraich ML, Lindgren S, Stromquist A, Milich R, Davis C, Watson D. Stimulant medication use by primary care physicians in the treatment of attention deficit hyperactivity disorder. Pediatrics 190;86:95–101.

19. Silver LB. The relationship between learning disabilities, hyperactivity, distractibility, and behavioral problems. J Am Acad Child Psychiatry 1981;20:285–297.

20. Shaywitz SE, Shaywitz BA. Attentional Deficit Disorder: Current Perspectives. In: Kavanaugh JF, Truss TJ, eds. Learning Disabilities: Proceedings of the National Conference. Parkton, MD: York Press, 1988.

21. August GJ, Holmes CS. Behavior and academic achievement in hyperactive subgroups and learning-disabled boys. Am J Dis Child 1984;138:1025–1029.

22. American Psychiatric Association. Diagnostic and Statistical Manual of Mental Disorders (3rd edition revised). Washington, DC: American Psychiatric Association, 1987.

23. Gittelman R, Mannuzza S. Diagnosing ADD-H in adolescents. Psychopharm Bull 1985;21:237–242.

24. Conners CK. Rating scales for use in drug studies for children. Psychopharm Bull 1974 (special issue);24–60.

25. Cohen ML, Kelly PC, Atkinson AW. Parent, teacher, child: a trilateral approach to attention deficit disorder. Am J Dis Child 1989;143:1229–1233.

26. Trites RL, Blouin AGA, Laprade K. Factor analysis of the Conners Teacher Rating Scale based on a large normative sample. J Counsel Clin Psychol 1982;50:615–623.

27. Brown RT, Borden MA, Clingerman SR. Pharmacotherapy in ADD adolescents with special attention to multimodality treatments. Psychopharm Bull 1985;21:192–211.

28. McBride MC. An individual double-blind crossover trial for assessing methylphenidate response in children with attention deficit disorder. J Pediatr 1988;113:137–145.

29. Klorman R, Brumaghim JT, Fitzpatrick PA, Borgstedt AD. Clinical effects of a controlled trial of methylphenidate on adolescents with attention deficit disorder. J Am Acad Child Adoles Psychiatry 1990;29:702–709.

30. Jacobvitz D, Sroufe LA, Stewart M, Leffert N. Treatment of attentional and hyperactivity problems in children with sympathomimetic drugs: a comprehensive review. J Am Acad Child Adoles Psychiatry 1990;29:677–688.

CHAPTER 15

Rationale and Recommendations: Infectious Diseases

PREVENTION STRATEGY

Although primary vaccination schedules are usually completed during earlier childhood, all adolescents will need booster vaccination for diphtheria and tetanus; some may need a second vaccination for measles, mumps and rubella to complete their primary series; and many sexually active adolescents will need vaccination for hepatitis B virus. GAPS recommendations for immunizations follow the guidelines developed by the Advisory Committee on Immunization Practices. Based on CDC guidelines, GAPS also recommends a selective strategy for screening adolescents for tuberculosis. Physicians are reminded that certain adolescents with chronic physical disorders and those who have had splenectomies may need influenza and pneumococcal vaccine. Screening for sexually transmitted diseases and for HIV infection are addressed in GAPS Recommendations 17 and 18, respectively. Physician guidelines for screening for tuberculosis are addressed in Recommendation 23, and guidelines for adolescent immunizations are addressed in Recommendation 24.

DISCUSSION

Measles, Mumps, and Rubella

Preventable infectious diseases such as measles, mumps, and rubella—usually considered threats to the health of younger children—can cause significant morbidity and mortality when contracted by adolescents and adults. Dramatic reductions over the past several decades in the number of cases of these three diseases resulted from the implementation of a universal immunization strategy. Recently, however, there has been renewed concern. Outbreaks of measles, mumps, and rubella continue to occur, even among populations previously vaccinated (1, 2). In addition, the number of cases of

Table 15.1. Reported Cases of Notifiable Diseases in 1991 by Age

Disease	Total Number of Cases	Age 10-14	Age 15-19	Age 20-24
Mumps	3,327	900 (27%)	639 (19%)	226 (15%)
Measles	9,593	900 (9%)	1096 (11%)	657 (7%)
Rubella	1,104	169 (15%)	191 (17%)	141 (8%)
Hepatitis B	17,435	207 (1%)	1337 (8%)	2719 (6%)
Tuberculosis	26,261	252 (1%)	601 (2.5%)	1370 (19%)

Source: Centers for Disease Control. Summary of notifiable diseases, United States 1991. MMWR 1992;40:1-63

these three diseases has recently increased, especially among older adolescents and those who are in institutional settings.

As shown in Table 15.1, 46% of all mumps cases, 20% of all cases of measles, and 32% of all cases of rubella reported in the United States during 1991 were among adolescents 10–19 years of age (3). Adolescents may be susceptible to these diseases for several reasons: (1) they did not receive the recommended vaccinations, (2) they received relatively ineffective vaccines, (3) they received appropriate vaccines but at too young an age, (4) they received incomplete immunizations regimens, or (5) they received vaccine by an inappropriate method (2).

Although monovalent vaccines are available for each virus (e.g., rubella, rubeola, mumps), the trivalent measles-mumps-rubella (MMR) is the choice for routine vaccination programs. Both the American Academy of Pediatrics (AAP) and the Advisory Committee on Immunization Practices (ACIP) of the Centers for Disease Control and Prevention recommend that all children receive two doses of MMR (2, 4). However, while the ACIP recommends that the second MMR be given at entry into elementary school, the AAP recommends that the vaccination be administered at entry into middle or junior high school. In relation to GAPS, the difference between the two sets of recommendations is moot—there is consensus that by the time of puberty all susceptible adolescents should have two doses of MMR. Thus, those who have not received their second dose during earlier childhood should be given this vaccination. Adverse reactions to MMR, even in previously immunized adolescents, are rare.

Hepatitis B Virus

Hepatitis B (HBV) is another preventable infectious disease that predominantly affects adolescents and young adults. As shown in Table 15.1, 9% of acute HBV infections reported to CDC during 1991 occurred in adolescents age 10–19 (3). These figures greatly underestimate the rate of hepatitis B infection, however, because it is not an officially reportable disease. Adjusting for under-reporting and including estimates for the proportion of infections that are asymptomatic, a better estimate is 200,000–300,000 HBV cases a year (5). Although 75% of people with HBV infection have subclinical infections, almost 3% will require hospitalization and 0.1% will die of fulminating disease (6). Of the estimated 750,000 to 1,000,000 people who are chronic carries of HBV, 25% will develop chronic hepatitis, which places them at high risk for cirrhosis or primary cancer of the liver.

Using data from a national sample of youth, McQuillan and associates have estimated the seroprevalence of HBV among adolescents 12–24 as 2.2 per 100 white youths and 4.7 per 100 black youths (7). Older adolescents have greater seroprevalence rates compared to younger adolescents. Among black youths, males have greater rates than do females, but there is no major gender difference among whites.

Transmission of HBV occurs through percutaneous or mucosal routes by sexual contact, use of contaminated needles, or from secretions infecting skin lesions or mucosal surfaces (8). The virus can also be transmitted to the newborn by passage through the birth canal. Transmission through blood transfusion can occur, but is rare. Because of the methods of transmission, it is not surprising that HBV is found with increased frequency among certain groups of adolescents, such as males engaging in sex with other males, heterosexuals with multiple partners, and users of illicit parenteral drugs. Alter and associates interviewed 1,917 people with acute hepatitis B infection, 63% of whom were between age 15 and 29 (9). Male homosexual activity was reported by 21%, parenteral drug use by 15%, heterosexual exposure by 18%, and various miscellaneous risk factors by 8%; 37% of people had no obvious risk factor for infection.

Immunization against HBV using recombinant DNA vaccine appears effective and safe (10). Recently, both the ACIP and the AAP revised their guidelines to recommend universal HBV vaccination for infants (8, 11). Although the new guidelines recommend that all adolescents who engage in behaviors that place them at risk for infection should be immunized, widespread use of HBV vaccine is also encouraged. The decision toward mass immunization was based on: (1) the serious morbidity resulting from the disease, (2) the lack of success with previous attempts to immunize only selected people who engage in behaviors that place them at high risk for the disease, and (3) the fact that 60% of adolescents and 30–40% of adults with acute hepatitis B infection do not have an identifiable risk factor (5, 8, 9, 12). The decision by ACIP and AAP to immunize all infants, but not all children, was made because of concern that there would be insufficient financial resources to implement a total universal primary prevention strategy.

Tuberculosis

The rates of tuberculosis (TB) fell between 1981 and 1988, then leveled off, and subsequently again began to rise (13, 14). In 1991, there were over 26,000 cases of TB, of which almost 3.5% occurred in youths 10–19 years old. Barry and associates studied the prevalence rate of a positive TB skin test among 2,799 students in Boston public schools and found that 5.1% of 7th graders and 8.9% of 10th graders were tuberculin positive (15). Although there were no differences in rates by gender, non-Hispanic white students had substantially lower rates than did other students. Nationally, over 60% of cases of tuberculosis occur among racial and ethnic minorities (16). The ratio of reported TB cases during 1987 was 5.7:1 for nonwhite adolescents compared to white adolescents age 15–24.

Although the association is unclear, the epidemic of HIV infections has contributed significantly to the rise in cases of TB. Thus, high rates of TB are noted predominantly in HIV epicenters (13, 14). Tuberculosis is also disproportionally encountered in people who are recent immigrants (13, 14, 16). The proportion of foreign born adolescents with tuberculosis has risen from 40% in 1986 to 49% in 1990 (14). In the study by Barry and associates, 87% of adolescents with a positive tuberculin test were born outside of the United States (15). Other groups with high rates of tuberculosis include people in correctional institutions and the homeless (14).

The Centers for Disease Control and Prevention, the U.S. Preventive Services Task Force, and the American Academy of Pediatrics recommend routine TB testing of populations at high risk for infection (17–18). This position is also adopted by GAPS. In addition, the AAP also recommends that children not at high risk for infection be screened for TB at three developmental stages—12—15 months, 4–6 years, and 14–16 years. GAPS leaves it to the discretion of the primary provider whether routine screening of low-risk adolescents should be performed.

Diphtheria and Tetanus

As a result of routine, universal immunization practices, diphtheria and tetanus have become uncommon infections. In 1991, there were only 5 cases of diphtheria and 57 cases of tetanus reported to the CDC, as compared to 1945 when there were 18,675 and over 500 cases of the two diseases, respectively (3). To maintain high levels of immunity, however, booster vaccinations after the initial childhood series are needed every 10 years (2). Reimmunization with pertussis is not necessary because the disease is relatively benign among adolescents (2).

CLINICAL APPLICATION

Adolescents should receive a second MMR vaccination if they: (1) have not had measles, mumps, or rubella infections documented by a physician; (2) lack laboratory evidence of immunity; or (3) have not had two doses of MMR vaccination. Immunization records of adolescents entering college, the military, or other institutional settings with dormitory living should be carefully reviewed, as should records of adolescents working in health care settings or in day care facilities. Preferably, the second MMR should be given during early puberty, prior to a time when the adolescent is at increased risk for pregnancy. Although a theoretical precaution, adolescents at risk for pregnancy should be cautioned about avoiding pregnancy for three months after vaccination.

Hepatitis B vaccination requires three doses administered approximately 1–2 months apart. As with MMR, this immunization series should be given during early puberty, or when there is an increase in the risk status of the adolescent. Risk status includes any adolescent who is sexually active or who lives in an area with a high prevalence of HIV and STD infections and unintended pregnancy. Widespread use of HBV vaccination is encouraged.

Testing for TB should be performed by a Mantoux test using five tuberculin units of purified protein derivative with a reading performed at 48–72 hours. Among adolescents who are at high risk for infection, induration of 10 mm or greater is considered positive. Adolescents with a positive test should be evaluated for active tuberculosis. The frequency of TB testing is left to the discretion of the physician. Adolescents with a positive test should be treated according to current standards of care as established by the CDC and by the AAP.

The diphtheria-tetanus booster should be administered 10 years after the previous immunization. Since the previous immunization usually occurred at 5–6 years of age, the booster should be given at age 15–16. This immunization should not include pertussis vaccine.

REFERENCES

1. Centers for Disease Control. Measles prevention: recommendations of the Advisory Committee on Immunization Practices (ACIP). MMWR 1989;38(S-9):1–18.

2. Committee on Infectious Disease. Report of the Committee on Infectious Disease: 1991. Elk Grove Village, IL: American Academy of Pediatrics, 1991.

3. Centers for Disease Control. Summary of notifiable diseases, United States 1991. MMWR 1992;40:1–63.

4. Centers for Disease Control. Rubella prevention: recommendations of the Immunization Practices Advisory Committee (ACIP). MMWR 1990;39(RR-15):1–20.

5. Margolis HS, Alter MJ, Hadler SC. Hepatitis B. Evolving epidemiology and implications for control. Semin Liver Dis 1991;11:84–92.

6. Centers for Disease Control. Protection against viral hepatitis. MMWR 1990;39(R-2):1–26.

7. McQuillan GM, Townsend TR, Fields HA. Seroepidemiology of hepatitis B in the United States: 1976 to 1980. Am J Med 1989;87(suppl 3A):5–10.

8. Centers for Disease Control. Hepatitis B Virus: a comprehensive strategy for eliminating transmission in the United States through universal childhood vaccination. MMWR 1991;40(RR-13):1–25.

9. Alter MJ, Hadler SC, Margolis HS. The changing epidemiology of hepatitis B in the United States: need for alternative vaccination strategies. JAMA 1990;263:1218–1222.

10. Andre FE, Path FRC. Summary of safety and efficacy data on a yeast-derived hepatitis B vaccine. Am J Med 1989;87(suppl 3A):14–20.

11. American Academy of Pediatrics, Committee on Infectious Diseases. Universal hepatitis B immunization. Pediatrics 1992;89:795–800.

12. Hall CB, Halsey NA. Control of hepatitis B: To be or not to be? Pediatrics 1992;90:274–277.

13. Jereb JA, Kelly GD, Dooley SW, Cauthen GM, Snider DE. Tuberculosis morbidity in the United States: final data, 1990. MMWR 1991;40(SS-3):23–27.

14. Starke JR, Jacobs RF, Jereb J. Resurgence of tuberculosis in children. J Pediatr 1992;120:839–855.

15. Barry MA, Shirley L, Grady MT, et al. Tuberculosis infection in urban adolescents: results of a school-based testing program. Am J Public Health 1990;80:439–441.

16. Snider DE, Salinas L, Kelly GD. Tuberculosis: an increasing problem among minorities in the United States. Pub Health Rep 1989;104:646–653.

17. Centers for Disease Control. A strategic plan for the elimination of tuberculosis in the United States. MMWR 1989;38(S-3):1–25.

18. US Preventive Services Task Force. Guide to Clinical Preventive Services. Baltimore: Williams & Wilkins, 1989.

CHAPTER 16

Delivery of Adolescent Preventive Services

Although some physicians provide many of the preventive services recommended by GAPS, and many physicians provide some of the services, comprehensive clinical preventive services are not currently a central component of adolescent health care (1). Reasons for this include uncertainty relating to the optimal periodicity and content of preventive care visits, questions about the importance and efficacy of preventive services in changing behavior, and inadequate reimbursement for preventive services (2, 3).

The body of evidence provided in *AMA Guidelines for Adolescent Preventive Services* should help to reduce the uncertainty about how frequently adolescents should be seen for preventive service visits, and what should be the content of these visits. The information presented in this book should also increase physicians' confidence that providing preventive services will have a beneficial effect on adolescent health. Another barrier to implementing preventive services—obtaining financial reimbursement more appropriate for the services delivered—is being addressed within the health care reform debate. The roles of prevention and adolescent preventive services are included in various health reform proposals, including the 1993 standard health benefits package proposed by the AMA.

The remainder of this chapter will address various considerations that may help promote use of GAPS in clinical settings, including a discussion of how GAPS services can be billed using the new and revised Current Procedural Terminology (CPT) codes, principles of health guidance, and the organization of the preventive service visit.

Coding and Reimbursement for Preventive Services

Reimbursement for preventive services varies depending on the insurance carrier and the individual patient contract. The Early and Periodic Screening Diagnosis and Treatment (EPSDT) program provides for annual preventive service visits for adolescents from low-income families. Managed care programs will also generally cover many preventive services, while indemnity insurance programs often cover only selected procedures. Because of the complexities involved in reimbursement for preventive services from private insurance companies, the remainder of this section will address changes in the CPT coding system that facilitate this process.

The 1993 edition of CPT has new codes for services essential to the delivery of GAPS recommendations: preventive services, counseling and/or risk reduction, and immunizations (4). The following points are necessary to understand how the new codes can be used for GAPS services (4–6):

1. CPT defines a "new" patient, distinct from an "established" patient, as someone ". . . who has not received professional services from the physician during the past three years" (4). For example, an adolescent first seen by a physician while hospitalized and then seen by the same physician in a ambulatory setting for an initial GAPS visit would be coded as an established patient for the outpatient service. On the other hand, an adolescent referred by the emergency room physician or by a physician who provided inpatient care would be coded as a new patient when seen for the initial GAPS visit.

2. In contrast to earlier editions, CPT now separates preventive care services into two categories: (1) preventive medicine services and (2) counseling and/or risk reduction services. Preventive medicine service codes should be used when ". . . services are preformed in the absence of patient complaints. The extent and focus of the service will largely depend on the age of the patient, the circumstances of the examination, and the abnormalities encountered" (4). For "new" adolescent patients, these codes would be 99383 for adolescents age 11, 99384 for those age 12–17, and 99385 for those age 18–21. Preventive medicine service codes for "established" adolescent patients are 99393 (11-year-olds), 99394 (12–17-year-olds), and 99395 (18–21-year-olds).

Physicians should remember that preventive medicine service codes pertain only to the time spent for the evaluation and management of asymptomatic patients. If symptoms or health problems are identified (e.g., use of tobacco or alcohol, unprotected sexual intercourse, high blood pressure, excessive weight loss) and a management plan developed, the office service codes should be used. In these situations, separate conditions identified during the visit should be classified according to The International Classification of Diseases, 9th Revision, Clinical Modification (ICD-9-CM) (7). Follow-up visits to further assess the identified problem would also then be charged using the office service codes. Because of closer scrutiny by health care payors, care must be taken to document in the adolescent's chart the nature of the symptoms or health problem.

3. Along with a preventive medicine code, an additional CPT code should be used if further time is spent with counseling and/or risk reduction activities. Counseling can be used to provide health guidance (e.g., anticipatory guidance) with the purpose of promoting health, and preventing injury and illness. These counseling codes—99401 to 99404—vary according to time (i.e., from 15 minutes to 60 minutes) spent with an adolescent.

These same counseling codes can conceivably be used when providing health guidance to parents. Health guidance provided in a group session has a code of 99411 for a 30-minute visit and 99412 for a 60-minute visit. Counseling and/or risk reduction service codes are used without distinction as to whether the adolescent is a "new" or "established" patient. As with the preventive medicine service codes, counseling codes can only be used with adolescents who have no identifiable symptom or health problem. Adolescents who receive brief office counseling targeting a specific health problem would receive an office service code, which includes a counseling component. When counseling or when coordination of care for a specific condition consumes more than 50% of the total time of the visit, documentation should be made in the adolescent's chart as to the exact time spent on these components, and the visit is coded based on time.

Because annual GAPS visits include both health guidance and screening, service codes for these visits may contain at least two designations—one for the preventive medicine service and another for counseling and/or risk reduction service. If additional time is spent providing health guidance to an adolescent's parents, then the physician has two options: (1) use a preventive care service code which relates to an extended counseling visit (e.g., 99412) combining the time spent with the adolescent and his or her parents or (2) use the modifier "-21" after the counseling code (99412) to designate that the service was greater than that usually provided for the higher level of service. Some insurers may not be accustomed to reimbursing for two CPT codes; consequently, physicians should alert local insurance carriers to their office practices and policies. Other CPT codes that can help with implementing GAPS services include the following:

- 99361 (30 minutes) or 99362 (60 minutes): These codes can be used for case management services in which the physician meets with a variety of other health professionals to plan or coordinate the adolescent's evaluation and treatment. To use this code, neither the adolescent nor the parent needs to be present.

- 99420: This code is used when a health-risk appraisal questionnaire is administered, or when the results of the appraisal are interpreted. The appraisal must be a standardized instrument administered either at or before the preventive service visit. Examples of instruments might include self-image questionnaires, depression inventories, eating disorder questionnaires, etc.

4. Care must be taken to use the CPT code that is specifically for the vaccination provided during adolescence. For example, the CPT code for the infant dose of diphtheria-tetanus is 90702, while the adult dose used during adolescence is 90718. The CPT code for the trivalent measles, mumps, rubella vaccination is 90707, and does not vary by age. Coding for the vaccination against hepatitis B (HBV)—90731—is complicated by the three different dose sizes of the vaccine. Infants receive the smallest dose of HBV. Children and younger adolescents receive the next size dose of HBV vaccine, while older adolescents usually receive the adult level of vaccine. Check with your local insurance carrier to determine its preference in reporting these services.

In general, there are two ways insurers can reimburse for immunizations (4). One method is for the immunization code to cover all the expenses associated with the immunization, including the cost of the vaccine, supplies (e.g., syringe), and administrative costs. The other method, used by some state Medicaid and some managed care organizations, is to reimburse only for the cost of the vaccine. With this method, administrative costs and supplies associated with providing the immunization are assumed included with the regular cost of the visit. Local carriers should be contacted to determine which method of reporting they prefer.

HEALTH GUIDANCE

Communicating with adolescents requires a special sensitivity to their stage of development and their cognitive abilities. Effective physician-adolescent and physician-parent communication is essential to screen and identify health problems, as well as to promote the adolescent's compliance with a recommended plan of action. Most adolescents are eager to talk about their health concerns with a physician, particularly if assured that the information will remain confidential. An assurance of confidentiality is especially important to this age group when sensitive topics such as sexual behavior, drug and alcohol use, and depression are discussed (8, 9).

Because providing factual information to adolescents requires less time than an interactive health guidance process, physicians often use this method of counseling when faced with busy clinic schedules. The results of various studies, however, suggest that providing information or advice alone is insufficient to promote behavioral change in adolescents (10–12). Health guidance is most effective when it is interactive, that is, when the adolescent and physician have an opportunity to listen to each other, express concerns about a particular issue, and jointly develop a plan of action to address those concerns (13, 14).

Agreement by the physician and adolescent on the nature of health concerns can have a positive effect on the clinical outcome. For example, Starfield and associates reviewed the medical records for 135 clinic visits of both adult and children patients (14). A total of 275 health problems were identified. The manner in which these problems were communicated to the patients was categorized, and then the association between these approaches and the patients' clinical outcomes were analyzed. Sixty-six percent of health problems identified by the physician alone showed little or no improvement at follow-up. By contrast, 60% of problems mutually agreed upon by both the physician and the patient showed improvement at follow-up, regardless of the perceived severity or the type of problem.

Health guidance should encourage adolescents to maintain healthy lifestyles and to develop social skills they can use to resist peer pressure and make appropriate decisions about their health behaviors. Techniques for improving the effectiveness of health guidance include the following:

1. Define with the adolescent the nature and extent of the health-risk behaviors that are problematic.
2. Determine the adolescent's attitude toward the behavior, his or her level of knowledge regarding possible consequences of the behavior, reasons for the behavior, and motivation to change.
3. Reinforce healthy behaviors and health promotion messages from school, family, and the community.
4. Determine with the adolescent a concrete, personalized course of action.
5. Encourage the adolescent to commit to this plan and provide positive reinforcement when success is achieved.

Health guidance can be delivered in a variety of ways, including personal counseling, brochures and other printed information, and audiovisual or computer-assisted messages. Health messages are most effective when they are reinforced within the office environment, and among the office and school, the family, and community organizations (15). For example, the absence of ashtrays in the office, antismoking posters and pamphlets in the waiting room, and health guidance messages during the clinical interview all reinforce an anti-tobacco message.

Organization of Preventive Services Visit

When first reviewing GAPS, physicians might think the recommendations are unrealistically time-consuming in light of the time demands of clinical practice. It is important, however, for physicians to recognize two points: first, GAPS organizes existing recommendations for clinical preventive services into a systematic approach directed at adolescents; until now, such recommendations were presented in a relatively haphazard fashion. Second, the entire complement of GAPS recommendations is not necessarily provided at each visit. For example, health guidance for parents is recommended only twice, while physical examinations for adolescents are recommended only three times. In addition, physicians may choose to emphasize various health guidance and screening recommendations, depending on the specific health characteristics of the population they service and on individual patient needs. The periodicity and content of recommended GAPS services are summarized in Table 16.1.

Table 16.1. Preventive Health Services by Age and Procedure

Procedure	Age of Adolescent										
	Early				Middle			Late			
	11	12	13	14	15	16	17	18	19	20	21
Health Guidance											
Parenting*		●				●					
Development	●	●	●	●	●	●	●	●	●	●	●
Diet and Fitness	●	●	●	●	●	●	●	●	●	●	●
Lifestyle**	●	●	●	●	●	●	●	●	●	●	●
Injury Prevention	●	●	●	●	●	●	●	●	●	●	●
Screening											
History											
Eating Disorders	●	●	●	●	●	●	●	●	●	●	●
Sexual Activity***	●	●	●	●	●	●	●	●	●	●	●
Alcohol and Other Drug Use	●	●	●	●	●	●	●	●	●	●	●
Tobacco Use	●	●	●	●	●	●	●	●	●	●	●
Abuse	●	●	●	●	●	●	●	●	●	●	●
School Performance	●	●	●	●	●	●	●	●	●	●	●
Depression	●	●	●	●	●	●	●	●	●	●	●
Risk for Suicide	●	●	●	●	●	●	●	●	●	●	●
Physical Assessment											
Blood Pressure	●	●	●	●	●	●	●	●	●	●	●
BMI	●	●		●	●		●	●		●	●
Comprehensive Exam		●			●			●			
Tests											
Cholesterol		1				1			1		
TB		2				2			2		
GC, Chlamydia, and HPV		3				3			3		
HIV and Syphilis		4				4			4		
Pap Smear		5				5			5		
Immunizations											
MMR		●									
Td						●					
HBV		6				6			6		

1. Screening test performed once if family history is positive for early cardiovascular disease or hyperlipidemia.
2. Screen if positive for exposure to active TB or lives/works in high-risk situation, (e.g., homeless shelter, jail, health care facility).
3. Screen at least annually if sexually active.
4. Screen if high-risk for infection.
5. Screen annually if sexually active or if 18 years or older.
6. Vaccinate if high-risk for hepatitis B infection.
* A parent health-guidance visit is recommended during early and middle adolescence.
** Includes counseling regarding sexual behavior and avoidance of tobacco, alcohol, and other drug use.
*** Includes history of unintended pregnancy and STD.

It is anticipated that most GAPS visits will last about 30 minutes, with somewhat more time needed for the initial visit. The basic components of all GAPS visits include the following:

Visit Orientation

Adolescents and their parents should be informed of the nature and purpose of each annual GAPS visit. This can be done with a reminder letter or postcard, by telephone, and/or upon arrival at the office.

Medical and Family History

At the initial GAPS visit, information about current health status, past medical history, and family history should be obtained. This information should be updated at each subsequent GAPS visit through use of a self-administered questionnaire, clinical interview, or a combination of both.

Adolescent Interview

Adolescents should be asked annually by the physician about current health concerns, as well as behaviors that may compromise health. These discussions should take place without the parent(s) present, and they should be confidential to ensure that adolescents discuss sensitive issues candidly.

Measurement Evaluation

All adolescents should have annual blood pressure, height, and weight measurements. The Body Mass Index (BMI), which is weight/height^2, should be used to determine the weight status of adolescents.

Management Plan

Information obtained from the history, clinical interviews, and physical examination should be used to develop a management plan. This plan might include the need for immunizations, laboratory tests, TB skin test, follow-up visits for further assessment, targeted counseling, treatment, or referral.

Health Guidance

GAPS recommends that all adolescents receive health guidance annually on growth and development, how to avoid health-risk behaviors, and how to prevent injuries. In addition, targeted counseling should be given to adolescent and parents, with specific needs as identified during the clinical visit.

In addition to the components described above, some GAPS visits will include the following:

Parent Interview

Parents should be interviewed alone at least once during early and middle adolescence to clarify past medical or family history, provide health guidance, and elicit parental concerns about the adolescent's health, behavior, and development.

Physical Examination

Adolescents should receive three complete physical examinations between age 11 and 21. Additional physical assessments should be done as warranted.

If, during the course of a preventive services visit, any physical, emotional, or behavioral problems are identified that appear to be an immediate health threat, physicians should use the remainder of the visit to focus on the acute problem. This shift in focus from prevention to intervention might include performing a pelvic examination to screen for a sexually transmitted disease, obtaining further history to assess risk of suicide, or determining the extent of immediate danger from alcohol or drug use. Alternatively, if the acute problems identified during the GAPS visit do not pose an immediate health threat, physicians should complete the preventive service agenda and ask the adolescent to return for further evaluation. Examples of problems that can wait until a later visit for more complete assessment include failing school grades, occasional alcohol use, smoking, and moderate weight loss.

REFERENCES

1. Igra V, Millstein SG. Current status and approaches to improving preventive services for adolescents. JAMA 1993;269:1408–1412.

2. US Preventive Services Task Force. Guide to Clinical Preventive Services: An Assessment of the Effectiveness of 169 Interventions. Baltimore: Williams & Wilkins, 1989.

3. Henry RC, Ogle KS, Snellman LA. Preventive medicine: physician practices, beliefs, and perceived barriers for implementation. Fam Med 1987;19:110–113.

4. Physicians' Current Procedural Terminology, 1993. Chicago: American Medical Association, 1992.

5. Suchyta RF, Ake J. Pediatric Procedural Terminology. Elk Grove Village, IL: American Academy of Pediatrics, 1992.

6. American Medical Association. Evaluation and management (E/M) codes for preventive services. CPT Assistant 1993;3:14–33.

7. The International Classification of Diseases (9th revision). Clinical Modification: ICD-9-CM (3rd edition). DHHS Publication No. (PHS) 89–1260. Washington, DC: US Department of Health and Human Services, 1989.

8. Malus M, LaChance P, Macauley A, Vanesse M. Priorities in adolescent health care: the teenagers' viewpoint. J Fam Pract 1987;25:159–162.

9. Erickson MP, Green LW, Fultz FG. Principles of changing health behavior. Cancer 1988;62:1768–1775.

10. Botvin G. Substance abuse prevention research: recent developments and future directions. J Sch Health 1986;56:369–374.

11. Flay B. Psychosocial approaches to smoking prevention: a review of findings. Health Psychol 1985;4:449–488.

12. Ockene J. Physician-delivered interventions for smoking cessation: strategies for increasing effectiveness. Prev Med 1987;16:723–737.

13. Emanuel EJ, Emanuel LL. Four models of the physician patient relationship. JAMA 1992;267:2221–2226.

14. Starfield B, Wray C, Hess K, Gross R, Birk PS, D'Lugoff BC. The influence of patient-practitioner agreement on outcome of care. Am J Public Health 1981;71:127–130.

15. Elster A, Panzarine S, Holt K. Proceedings from the AMA State of the Art Conference on Adolescent Health Promotion. Washington, DC: National Clearinghouse on Maternal and Child Health, 1993.

Key Characteristics of GAPS Recommendations

Target Conditions

GAPS addresses conditions that are amenable to primary and secondary preventive interventions. They were selected because of the burden of suffering caused by the conditions (i.e., prevalence of the condition, morbidity, and mortality) and because the conditions present the opportunity to effect change, prevent disease, and promote health.

Target Population

GAPS is directed at relatively healthy adolescents between the ages of 11 and 21. Several of the recommendations are intended for parents or adult caregivers of adolescents as well. GAPS recommendations are not intended as treatment guidelines for adolescents with identified health conditions.

Interventions

GAPS directs recommendations toward the following strategies:

1. Health Guidance. Both anticipatory guidance and health counseling are directed at the adolescent and/or parent. It can be provided by any qualified office staff and can consist of visual aids; interpersonal communication; or written, audiovisual, or computer-assisted material.
2. Screening. The identification of signs, symptoms, or precursors of the condition by use brief self-report questionnaire, computer-assisted interview, clinical interview, physical examination, and laboratory test. Screening, if positive, leads to further assessment and evaluation of the condition. GAPS does not include recommendations for diagnostic assessment.
3. Immunizations. Routine vaccination for the prevention of infectious diseases, such as rubella, rubeola, tetanus, diphtheria, mumps, and hepatitis B.

Providers and Setting

GAPS recommendations are intended for primary providers who see adolescents in ambulatory settings, including private offices and public medical clinics, school health centers, and community clinics. Primary care providers may include physicians, as well as those who work with physicians in the primary care setting, including nurses, health educators, and other allied health professionals.

Admissible Evidence

A hierarchy of strength of evidence was used in the review of information justifying GAPS recommendations. Level 1 information consists of data from experimental trials; Level 2 information consists of data from cohort or epidemiological studies; Level 3 information consists of recommendations from other major organizations or panels of experts. Case reports and descriptive studies from outside North America and Western Europe were excluded. To determine the relevance of the information for GAPS, the health care situation (i.e., adolescents seen in primary care settings), the setting of the study (i.e., community, school, office or clinic), and the sample studied (i.e., adolescents or adults) were noted for each piece of literature reviewed. Scientific literature for each condition was identified by soliciting articles from experts in the specified areas, conducting a computer search of the medical and social science literature dating from 1980 through 1991, and identifying key references prior to 1980 cited in articles reviewed.

Evaluation of the Evidence

AMA staff analyzed relevant research for each targeted condition and abstracted the findings. Charts were developed to delineate the articles or reports used, the level of scientific evidence, the setting, the sample size, and the age of subjects for each condition. Where abundant literature existed for a particular condition, selected articles were used, especially reports that related directly to adolescents. Supporting evidence for each condition included the following:

1. Burden of suffering: including a discussion of the epidemiology of the condition, the short-term and long-term consequences of the condition, and the risk factors for the condition.
2. Justification: including a discussion of the efficacy in identifying the target condition and the efficacy of preventive interventions.

The recommendations for each condition were then rated according to the strength of the supporting evidence. It is important to note that GAPS recommendations are justified by varying strengths of scientific information.

Review of Existing Organizational and Federal Policy

Health policies from national health organizations and recommendations from key reports of federal agencies, foundations, and commissions were identified, reviewed, and abstracted. This information was used as Level 3 evidence supporting GAPS recommendations.

Appropriateness of the Recommendations

An 11-person multidisciplinary Scientific Advisory Board provided advice on the development of GAPS. This Board included experts from the areas of pediatric and adolescent medicine, psychiatry, health and developmental psychology, health education, and preventive medicine. Consultation was also provided by a representative of the health insurance industry and an expert in adolescent medicine screening procedures. Direction and leadership for the Board was provided by an Executive Committee consisting of a health psychologist, a pediatrician, and AMA staff. The Scientific Advisory Board met once during 1990, twice during 1991, and once during 1992. Members reviewed the abstracted material to develop general, but unofficial, group consensus for each condition.

To ensure that the views of medical practitioners were appropriately considered, representatives of the following primary care medical groups participated on the GAPS national scientific advisory board:

> American Academy of Child and Adolescent Psychiatry
> American Academy of Pediatrics
> American Academy of Family Physicians
> American College of Obstetricians and Gynecologists
> American College of Physicians
> American Psychiatric Association
> Society for Adolescent Medicine

Input from other medical and nonmedical health professional organizations was solicited from the 32 organizations participating in the AMA National Coalition on Adolescent Health. Review of GAPS recommendations was also provided by a broad array of national organizations, the Public Health Service, and experts in child and adolescent health, advocacy, and health policy.

INDEX

Page numbers in italics denote figures; those followed by "t" denote tables.

A